PRACTICAL MANUAL ON
ORAL HISTOLOGY AND
ORAL PATHOLOGY

PRACTICAL MANUAL ON ORAL HISTOLOGY AND ORAL PATHOLOGY

Alka Dive
MDS
Professor and Head
Department of Oral and Maxillofacial Pathology
VSPM Dental College and Research Centre
Nagpur (Maharashtra)
INDIA

ELSEVIER

ELSEVIER

RELX India Pvt. Ltd.
Registered Office: 818, Indraprakash Building, 8th Floor, 21, Barakhamba Road, New Delhi-110001
Corporate Office: 14th Floor, Building No. 10B, DLF Cyber City, Phase II, Gurgaon-122002, Haryana, India

Notice

Practitioners and researchers must always rely on their own experience and knowledge in evaluating and using any information, methods, compounds or experiments described herein. Because of rapid advances in the medical sciences, in particular, independent verification of diagnoses and drug dosages should be made. To the fullest extent of the law, no responsibility is assumed by Elsevier, authors, editors or contributors for any injury and/or damage to persons or property as a matter of products liability, negligence or otherwise, or from any use or operation of any methods, products, instructions, or ideas contained in the material herein.

Manager, Content Strategy: Nimisha Goswami
Content Project Manager: Anand K Jha
Sr Graphic Designer: Milind Majgaonkar
Sr Production Executive: Ravinder Sharma

Laser typeset by GW India
Printed in India by EIH Limited-Unit Printing Press, IMT Manesar, Gurugram, Haryana.

Dedicated to
My Beloved Parents

Dr V W Kant
Dr (Mrs) Ashalata V Kant

Dr S G Dive
Mrs Shalini S Dive

Foreword

I take immense pleasure in writing a few words about the book *Practical Manual on Oral Histology and Oral Pathology* by Dr Alka Dive (Prof and Head), Department of Oral and Maxillofacial Pathology, VSPM Dental College and Research Centre, Nagpur. This book is an outcome of hardwork and sheer determination.

The most important aspect of this book is hand drawn diagrams (histology of oral and dental tissues and histopathology of oral lesions) with descriptions. Characteristic features are highlighted. Introduction of sample viva voce questions with answers is a very helpful addition for students to excel in practical examinations. This book is designed in a very simplified manner and thus makes the subject easy for understanding.

The oral and maxillofacial pathologist attempts to understand oral disease so that it can be properly diagnosed and adequately treated. The final diagnosis is based on histopathological examination, hence the need to understand the subject.

This book will definitely be useful to students primarily for the preparation of practical records. Dr Alka Dive deserves a word of appreciation for her sincere and painstaking effort. I am very sure that this book will be of great help to students

Dr Abid Biviji
Former Dean, Govt Dental College and Hospital, Nagpur
Sharad Pawar Dental College and Hospital, Sawangi (Meghe) Wardha
VSPM Dental College and Research Centre, Nagpur
Ex Director VSPM Dental College and Research Centre, Nagpur

Preface

Practical Manual on Oral Histology and Oral Pathology intends to provide students a diagrammatic overview of histological and histopathological features. It is a basic guide aimed at helping students to draw well labelled diagrams of oral histology and oral pathology in practical records and also to develop the interest of students in these subjects. The book covers majority of the topics from the undergraduate syllabus with descriptions of histological and histopathological features of each diagrams. Hand drawn diagrams with captions are for better understanding and also to ease drawing the diagrams. Characteristic features have been highlighted in each chapter.

This book is also equipped with some viva questions with answers for oral histology and oral pathology with answers. Oral pathology section of the book contains viva questions pertaining only to histopathological features. These viva voce questions with answers are a prototype and a guide to the most likely questions that can be asked during practical examination. Students are advised to read the concerned textbook in detail.

The diagrams are solely for understanding purpose, however some subjectivity in drawing these can be expected. I have tried my best to utilize my knowledge and experience in the subject while completing this book for the benefit of students.

Alka Dive

Acknowledgements

First and foremost I would like to thank the very dynamic publishing team of Elsevier India for bringing this book to a reality. I would like to express my gratitude towards Ms Shabina Nasim, Head, Content Project Management, Ms Nimisha Goswami, Manager, Content Strategy, and Mr Anand K Jha, Content Project Manager for good communication and timely cooperation. I am thankful to the Mr Sandeep Tomar for digitizing hand drawn diagrams and Mr Milind Majgaonkar for working on cover design.

I am forever indebted to my Guide Dr Biviji Sir and my teachers Dr V K Hazarey Sir and Dr Mrs S M Ganvir Madam for their able guidance throughout.

I am grateful to Dr Samantha Thakur for helping me to develop my ideas during the initial stages of this work. I would acknowledge Dr Shrutal Deshmukh in rigorously going through my work. I express my sincere thanks to my valued colleague and friend Dr Minal Chaudhari for always being there. My deep appreciation is due towards Dr Akshay Dhobley for his suggestions and help whenever required. I am thankful to my colleagues in the department, Dr Shubhangi Khandekar, Dr Ashish Bodhade, Dr Rohit Moharil and Dr Neena Dongre along with the post-graduate students for their constant support. I am also thankful to Dr Usha Radke, Dean of my college for her support.

This book would not have been possible without my strongest support system, i.e. my Family, whose love and guidance is always with me in everything I pursue. My deepest thanks to my relatives and well-wishers for their love and encouragement.

I thank every single person who has contributed towards completion of this book and beg forgiveness if I have failed to mention any of those names.

Lastly I thank the Almighty for making the endeavour possible.

Preparation of Specimen for Microscopic Examination

Histology means the study of microscopic structure of tissues and histopathology means microscopic examination of tissues in order to study the manifestations of disease. This requires the preparation of tissue for various types of microscopy. Routine histologic technique involves use of light microscopy (optical microscopy) in which focused light and lenses are used to magnify the specimen. The laboratory techniques are modified according to the type of specimen and type of microscopy used for the examination of specific or particular structures.

PREPARATION OF SOFT TISSUE SPECIMEN

Preparation of soft tissue specimen like gingiva, tongue, lips, cheeks for light microscopic examination involves:

- Fixation
- Dehydration
- Clearing
- Infiltration with wax
- Embedding
- Cutting the section
- Staining the section.

After careful removal of the tissue specimen, it should be immediately placed in fixing solution. Most common fixative is 10% neutral formalin. Fixation is done to coagulate the proteins and thus to reduce the alterations by subsequent laboratory procedures and to prevent autolysis. Period of fixation varies from several hours to days depending on the size of specimen and type of fixative used.

The specimen is washed overnight in running water after fixation in formalin. The specimen is gradually dehydrated in increasing percentage of alcohol, i.e. 40%, 60%, 80%, 95% alcohol to remove the water content from the specimen.

After dehydration, clearing is done in xylene which is the most commonly used clearing agent to remove the alcohol and to make the specimen ready for impregnation with wax.

The specimen is then infiltrated with wax, paraffin wax is routinely used medium for histology. The specimen is placed in melted paraffin wax. The temperature depends on the melting point of paraffin wax used and the time depends on the size and density of the specimen. All the xylene in the tissue is to be replaced by paraffin wax.

After complete infiltration with paraffin wax, the specimen is embedded in the block of paraffin. Two L- shaped metallic pieces of brass or aluminium are used to make a block and are kept on a metallic platform. The block is filled with melted paraffin. Then the specimen infiltrated with paraffin is placed in the block with proper orientation (the surface to be cut is facing downwards). The paraffin wax is allowed to harden.

The specimen is thus ready for section cutting on microtome. The paraffin block with specimen is clamped on a microtome. The microtome is adjusted to cut the sections of desired thickness (usually of 4 to 6 μm). The microscopic glass slides are covered with a thin film of Meyer's albumin adhesive and suitable lengths of paraffin ribbon are mounted on these slides. This is done by floating a paraffin ribbon in a pan of warm water and then prepared slide is slipped under the ribbon and lifted with ribbon from water which has tissue section of the specimen on the top. The slide is then allowed to dry on the drying table.

The slide is now ready for the staining. Most routinely used stain is haematoxylin and eosin (H & E). The stained tissue section is mounted with mountant (DPX the most commonly used mountant) and coverslip is fixed. As the mounting medium hardens, slides can be examined under the microscope.

In H& E stained sections, haematoxylin being a basic dye stains acidic structures like nucleus and eosin being an acidic dye has affinity for basic structures and thus stains cytoplasm.

Results

Nuclei – Blue
Cytoplasm, collagen, keratin, muscle – Pink
RBCs – Orange/**red**

PREPARATION OF HARD TISSUE SPECIMEN

The hard (calcified) tissues like teeth and bone studied by routine H & E stain. These hard tissues cannot be cut with microtome knife. Thus these are made soft by decalcification. The method is as follows:

After removal the specimen is fixed in fixative i.e. 10% neutral formalin.

After fixation, decalcification is done in decalcifying fluids like 5% nitric acid, formic acid, ethylene diamine tetraacetic acid (EDTA) etc. It may take few days to several weeks' time depending on the decalcifying agent used. Complete decalcification can be assessed by the 'feel' or by piercing the tissue carefully with a needle otherwise it may damage it or by taking radiograph or by chemical methods.

When decalcification is complete, the specimen is washed in running water for 24 hours to remove acid.

The next processing is same as done in processing of soft tissue.

Dentin, cementum and pulp tissue of tooth can be studied by this method except enamel as enamel is highly calcified structure, lost during the process of decalcification.

PREPARATION OF GROUND SECTION

Calcified structures like bone and teeth can also be studied under ground section. Tooth enamel being highly mineralized (96%), is lost during decalcification process. Thus undecalcified teeth and bone may be studied by preparation of ground section (GS).

For preparation of ground section of tooth, tooth to be kept in 10% neutral formalin until used. The tooth is ground down on a lathe by using coarse wheel first and then fine abrasive wheel with a continuous flow of water directed on the rotating wheel. After this it can be ground on an abrasive stone like Arkansas stone till the desired thickness is achieved (approx. 25 – 30 microns). This section is then dehydrated in increasing grades of alcohol, clearing is done in xylene to remove the alcohol and mounted on a glass slide with a mounting medium using DPX and covered with coverslip.

Enamel, dentin and cementum can be studied under the ground section of tooth.

Contents

ORAL HISTOLOGY

Development of Tooth 1

When the embryo is about 6 weeks old, the oral epithelium thickens and invaginates into the underlying ectomesenchyme along the horse shoe–shaped future dental arches. This leads to formation of primary epithelial band. By the 7th week, the primary epithelial band divides into buccally (outer) located vestibular lamina and lingually (inner) located dental lamina. The dental lamina contributes to development of teeth and is primordium for ectodermal portion of teeth. Tooth developmental stages are Bud stage, Cap stage and Bell stage according to the shape of enamel organ (epithelial part of tooth germ).

BUD STAGE

In the bud stage (Fig. 1.1), the *enamel organ* consists of *low columnar cells* which are placed *peripherally* and *polygonal cell* which are placed *centrally*. The *ectomesenchymal condensation* immediately adjacent to enamel organ is *dental papilla*. The *condensed ectomesenchyme surrounding enamel organ and dental papilla* is *dental sac*.

CAP STAGE

Unequal growth in different parts of the tooth bud and a shallow mesenchymal invagination on the deep surface of bud leads to formation of the cap stage. In the cap stage (Fig. 1.2), the enamel organ consists of:

i. *Peripheral cells* which are *cuboidal* and covering the *convexity of the cap* called *outer enamel (dental) epithelium.*
ii. *Inner layer of cells* which are *tall columnar* and covering the *concavity of cap* called *inner enamel (dental) epithelium.*
iii. *Polygonal cells* located in the centre of the enamel organ, i.e. the cells between the outer enamel epithelium and inner enamel epithelium, *become separated* and these polygonal cells

3

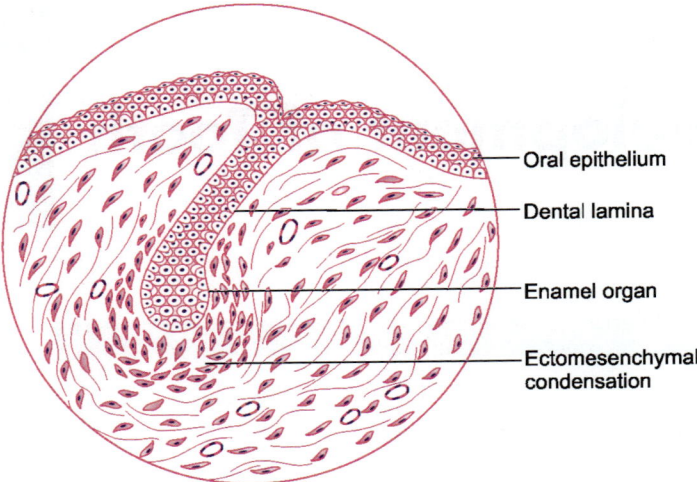

Figure 1.1 Bud stage – enamel organ and ectomesenchymal condensation (Ectomesenchyme – embryonic connective tissue derived from neural crest).

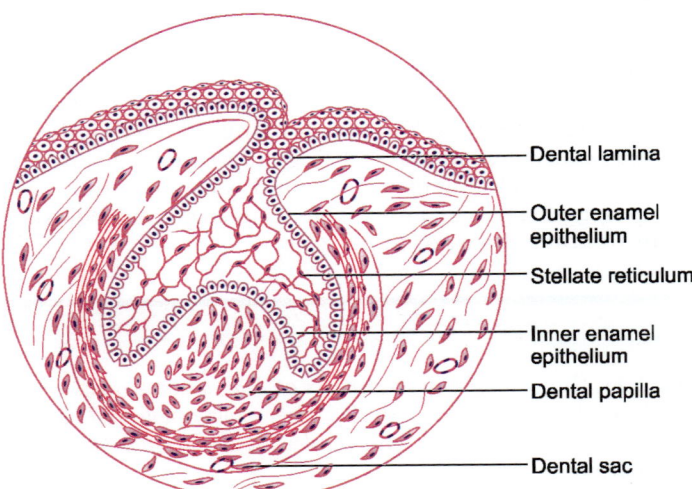

Figure 1.2 Cap stage – enamel organ consisting of outer enamel epithelium (cuboidal cells), stellate reticulum and inner enamel epithelium (tall columnar cells). Dental papilla and dental sac are seen.

become *star shaped* which form a *cellular network* and are called as *stellate reticulum*. It has a *cushion-like consistency* and acts as a *shock absorber* to support and protect delicate enamel-forming cells.

The condensed ectomesenchyme in the invaginated portion of inner enamel epithelium is called *dental papilla,* which *forms dentin and pulp.* Marginal condensation of ectomesenchyme surrounding enamel organ and dental papilla becomes more fibrous and is called *dental sac.* The outer enamel epithelium is separated from the dental sac and the inner enamel epithelium is separated from dental papilla by a basement membrane.

BELL STAGE

The invagination of epithelium deepens and continuous growth of enamel organ at its margins leads to formation of bell stage. In the bell stage (Fig. 1.3), the enamel organ consists of:

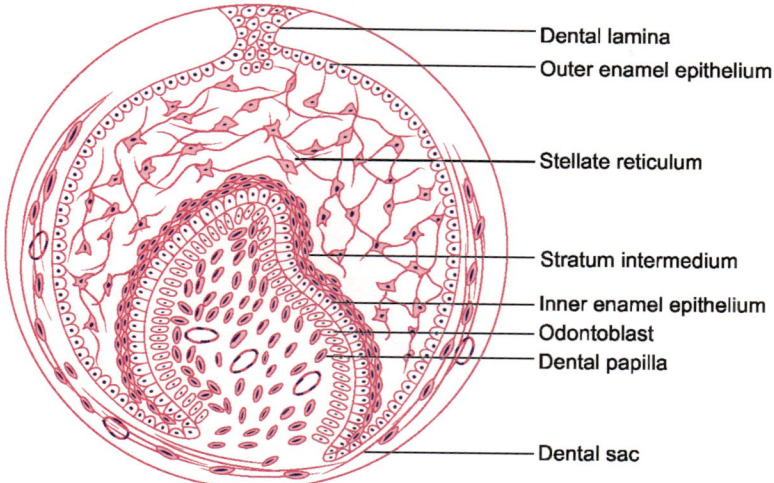

Figure 1.3 labels:
- Dental lamina
- Outer enamel epithelium
- Stellate reticulum
- Stratum intermedium
- Inner enamel epithelium
- Odontoblast
- Dental papilla
- Dental sac

Figure 1.3 Bell stage – enamel organ assumes a shape like a bell and consists of outer enamel epithelium, stellate reticulum, stratum intermedium and inner enamel epithelium. Dental papilla and dental sac are seen.

i. Outer layer of single row of cuboidal cells, i.e. *outer enamel epithelium.*
ii. Star-shaped cells with long processes which anastomose with adjacent cells, i.e. *stellate reticulum.*
iii. Two to three layers of flattened (squamous) cells between stellate reticulum and inner enamel epithelium, i.e. stratum intermedium which seems to be *essential for enamel formation.*
iv. Inner single layer of columnar cells, i.e. *inner enamel epithelium.*

The mesenchyme enclosed in the invaginated portion of enamel organ is *dental papilla.* Under the organizing influence of cells of inner enamel epithelium, the peripheral cells of dental papilla become cuboidal and later columnar, which are called *odontoblasts* (formative cells of dentin). The basement membrane separating the enamel organ and dental papilla is called membrana preformativa, which is future dentinoenamel junction.

The *dental sac* shows a *circular arrangement of fibres* and *forms a capsular structure.* This gives rise to the *formation* of *cementum, periodontal ligament* and *alveolar bone.*

There is degeneration of dental lamina and the enamel organ loses its connection with oral epithelium. *Remnants of dental lamina* are called *cell rests of Serres* which are discrete clusters of epithelial cells.

ADVANCED BELL STAGE

Advanced bell stage is characterized by *formation of hard dental tissues and root formation* (Fig. 1.4). The formation of dentin by odontoblasts always occurs first as a layer along the future dentinoenamel junction in the region of future cusps and then proceeds pulpally and apically. After the first layer of dentin has been laid down, the cells of the inner enamel epithelium

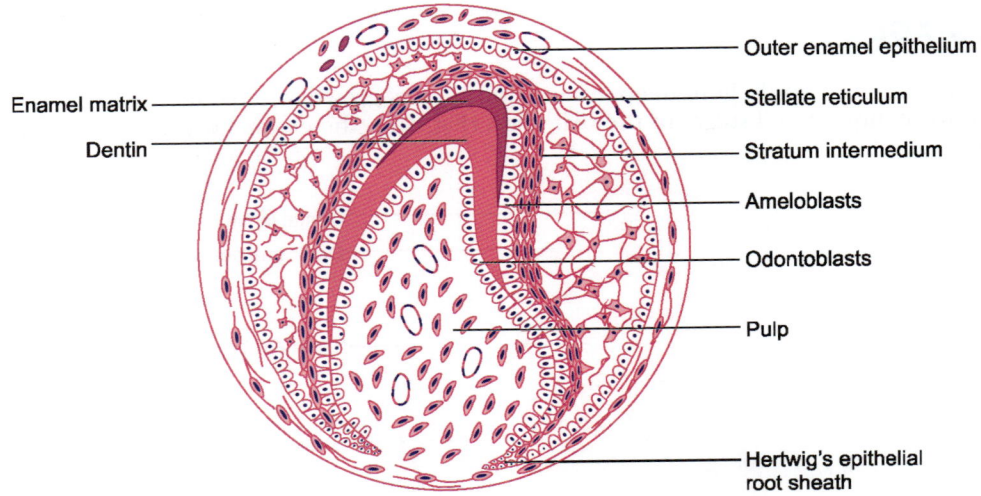

Figure 1.4   Advanced bell stage – formation of hard dental tissues and Hertwig's epithelial root sheath consisting of outer enamel epithelium and inner enamel epithelium.

differentiate into ameloblasts, which lay down enamel over the dentin in future incisal and cuspal area and then proceeds coronally and cervically.

In addition, *cervical portion of enamel organ* forms *Hertwig's epithelial root sheath* which *outlines the future root* and consists of *outer enamel epithelium and inner enamel epithelium.*

HERTWIG'S EPITHELIAL ROOT SHEATH: DEVELOPMENT OF ROOT

Root formation starts after enamel and dentin formation has reached future cementoenamel junction. Hertwig's epithelial root sheath (Fig. 1.5) consists of outer enamel epithelium and

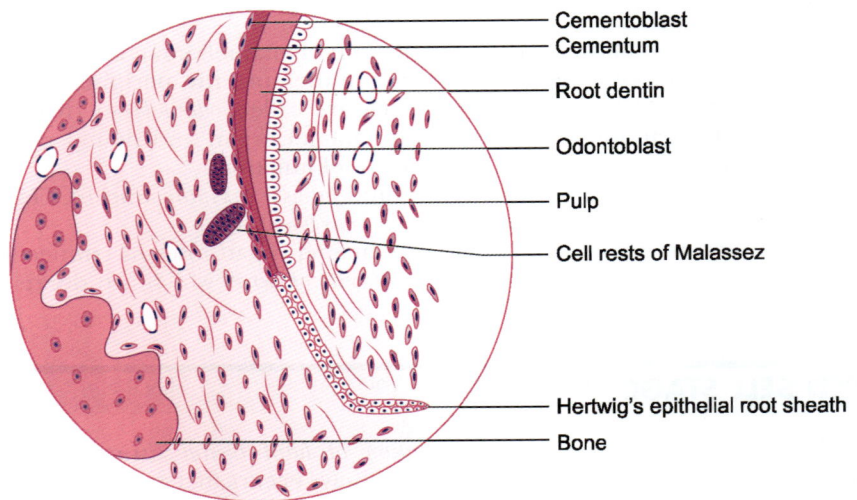

Figure 1.5   Hertwig's epithelial root sheath – root formation occurs from Hertwig's epithelial root sheath.

inner enamel epithelium (with no stratum intermedium and stellate reticulum). The cells of inner layer are short and do not produce enamel. These cells induce the differentiation of cells of radicular dental papilla into odontoblasts which form the first layer of root dentin. At the same time, the root sheath is broken and *its remnants* persist as small epithelial strands or clumps in periodontal ligaments as *cell rests of Malassez.* Coronal part of the sheath degenerates while apical part continues to grow in length and there is lengthening of root. The cells of dental sac differentiate into cementoblasts which lay down cementum over the root dentin.

Enamel | 2

ENAMEL RODS AND CROSS-STRIATIONS

The enamel consists of *enamel rods or prisms, rod sheaths and interprismatic substance* (Fig. 2.1). In longitudinal section, these enamel rods *run outward from the dentinoenamel junction towards the surface of the tooth*. Usually these rods are *perpendicular to the dentinoenamel junction*, run in *oblique direction and have a wavy course*. Each enamel rod shows *periodic bands* at *about 4-micron* interval which are *cross-striations* and these cross-striations demarcate rod segments. These appear as dark lines so as to have a *striated appearance*. These cross-striations are supposed to be due to diurnal rhythm in rod formation. In permanent teeth, the rods are directed apically in cervical region where as in deciduous teeth, the rods are parallel to occlusal surface, i.e. approximately horizontal.

INCREMENTAL LINES OF RETZIUS

Incremental lines of Retzius represent the *successive apposition of layers of enamel* during crown formation (Fig. 2.2). They appear as *dark brownish lines* in ground section of enamel. In longitudinal section, they run *from dentinoenamel junction toward the tooth surface*, deviating occlusally. In cervical parts of crown, they run obliquely. In transverse section, they appear as concentric circles like the rings of a tree.

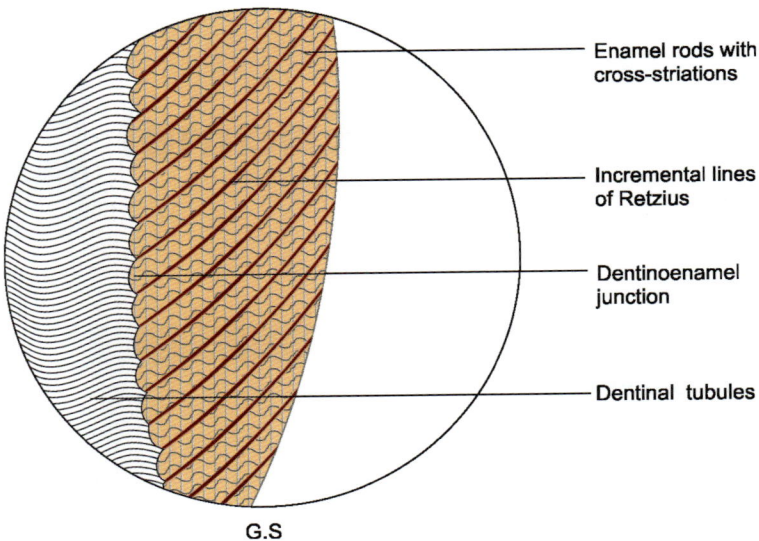

G.S

Figure 2.1 Enamel rods and cross-striations – enamel rods with cross-striations running outward from dentinoenamel junction towards the surface of the tooth.

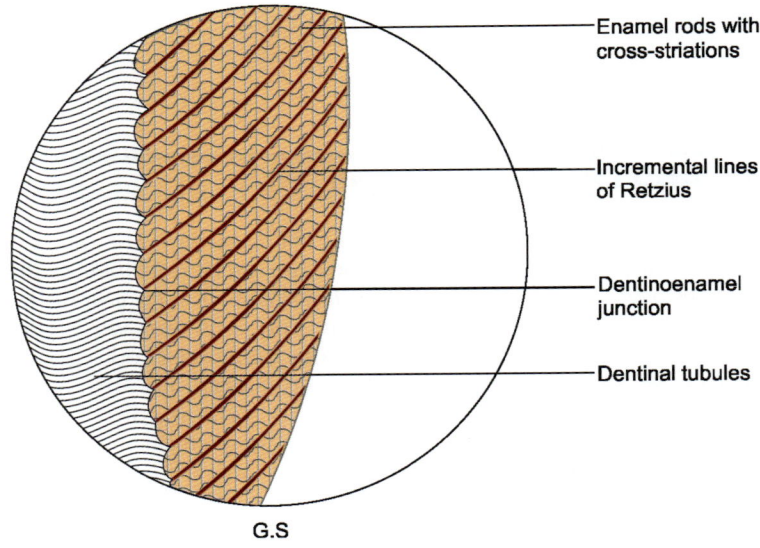

G.S

Figure 2.2 Incremental lines of Retzius – incremental lines of Retzius appearing as dark brownish lines representing the successive apposition of layers of enamel.

NEONATAL LINE

In deciduous teeth and first permanent molars, the enamel develops partly before birth (*prenatal enamel*) and partly after birth (*postnatal enamel*).This prenatal enamel is separated from postnatal enamel by an *accentuated incremental line of Retzius* which is referred as neonatal line or neonatal ring. It reflects the abrupt change in the environment and nutrition of the newborn infant. The

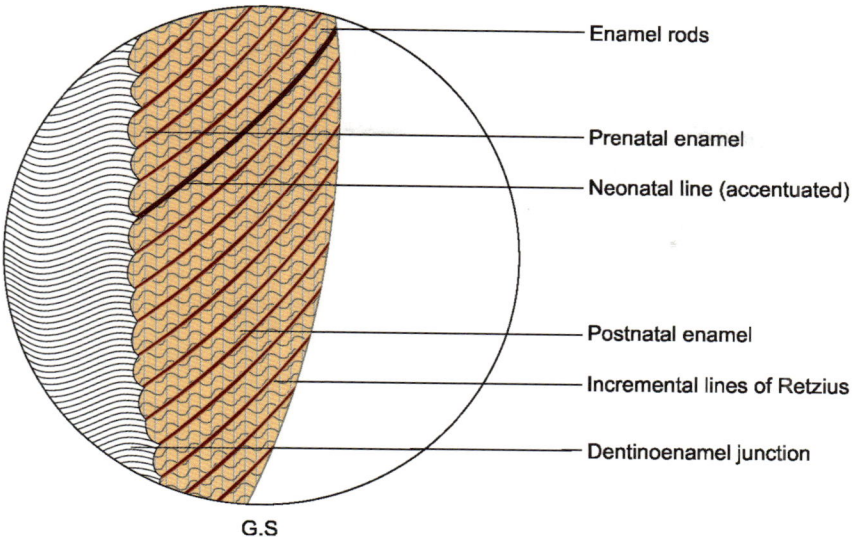

G.S

Figure 2.3   Neonatal line – neonatal line separating prenatal and postnatal enamel.

prenatal enamel is *better developed* than postnatal enamel as fetus develops in well protected environment with adequate supply of all essential materials (Fig. 2.3).

DENTINOENAMEL JUNCTION

The *junction between dentin and enamel* appears as a scalloped line, with the *convexities* of these scallops *towards the dentin* (Fig. 2.4). Rounded projections of the enamel fit into the shallow

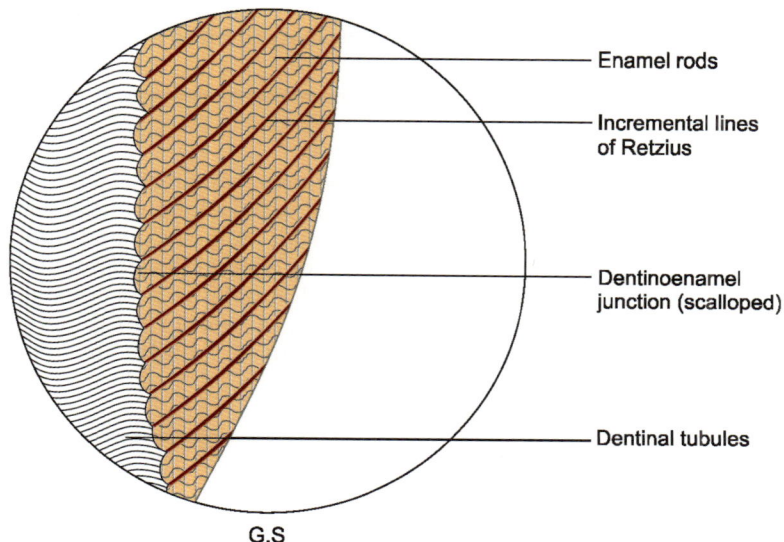

G.S

Figure 2.4   Dentinoenamel junction – the junction between dentin and enamel appears as scalloped line with convexities towards dentin.

depressions of dentin which cause *firm hold of enamel and dentin*. It can be seen in the arrangement of the ameloblasts and the basement membrane of the dental papillae and is preformed before the development of hard tissue.

ENAMEL TUFTS

Enamel tufts are seen to be arising *from dentinoenamel junction* for a short distance *into the enamel* (Fig. 2.5).They are narrow ribbon-like structures with the inner end at the dentin. As they *resemble a tuft of grass* when seen in ground sections they are termed as enamel tufts. They *follow the direction of enamel rods*. Enamel tufts *consist of hypocalcified enamel rods and interprismatic substance*.

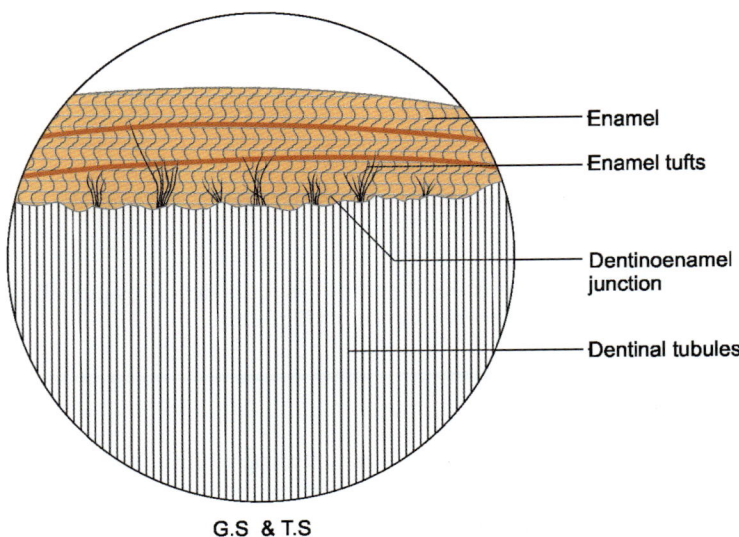

G.S & T.S

Figure 2.5   Enamel tufts – enamel tufts resembling tufts of grass and arising from dentinoenamel junction.

ENAMEL SPINDLES

Sometimes *odontoblastic processes of dentin cross the dentinoenamel junction and extend into enamel*. These are *most common beneath the cusp tip regions* and best seen in longitudinal sections of enamel. These structures do not follow the direction of enamel rods. Some of the odontoblastic processes extend into enamel epithelium during the early stages of enamel development and result in the formation of enamel spindles. The direction of the odontoblastic processes and spindles is at right angle to the surface of dentin. These are *hypocalcified structures* in the enamel. In ground sections of teeth, due to disintegration of organic content of spindles and replacement by air, these spaces *appears dark* in transmitted light (Fig. 2.6).

ENAMEL LAMELLAE

Enamel lamellae are *hypomineralized structures* that *extend from the enamel surface towards the dentinoenamel junction* or sometimes may penetrate into the dentin (Fig. 2.7). In ground sections, they *appear as thin, leaf-like structures* and narrower, longer and less common than enamel tufts. Enamel

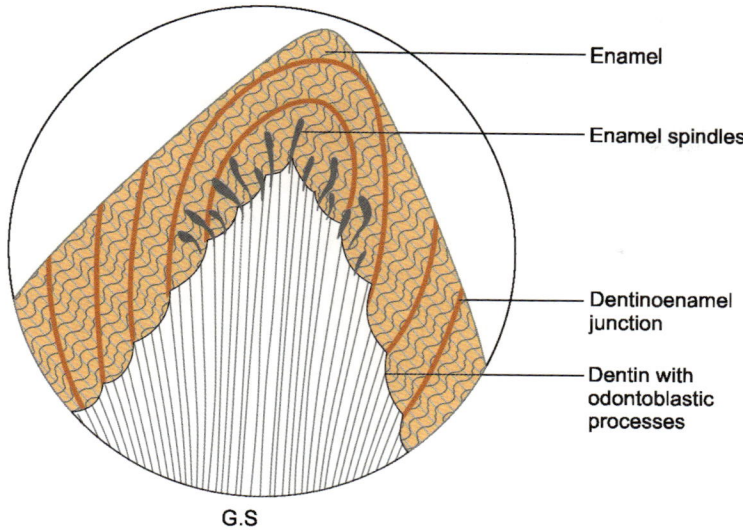

G.S

Figure 2.6   Enamel spindles – odontoblastic processes extending into enamel as enamel spindles.

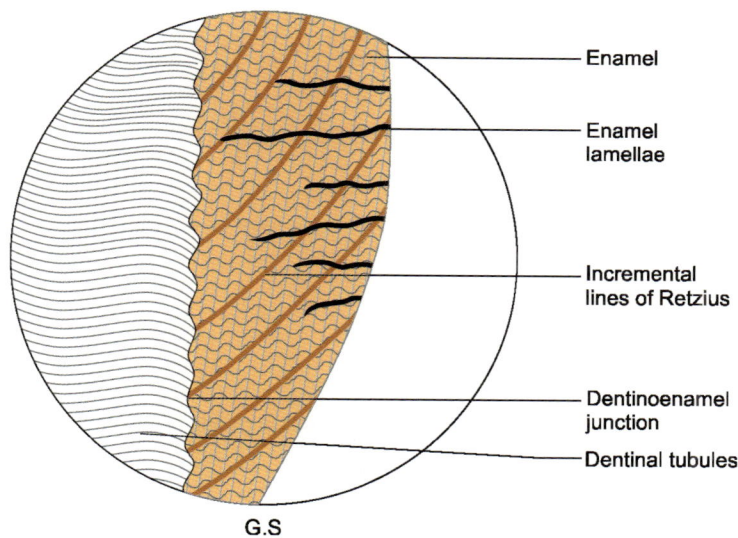

G.S

Figure 2.7   Enamel lamellae — enamel lamellae extending from enamel surface towards the dentinoenamel junction.

lamellae may be formed during the development due to incomplete maturation of groups of prisms or after eruption as cracks.

Enamel lamellae may be of three types:

Type A: composed of poorly calcified rod segments and seen in enamel.
Type B: composed of degenerated cells and may reach into dentin.
Type C: arising in erupted teeth where cracks are filled with organic matter derived from saliva, and may reach into dentin.

It has been suggested that enamel lamellae represent the defects in enamel and may provide entry to caries producing microorganisms.

HUNTER–SCHREGER BANDS

In longitudinal ground section of tooth under oblique reflected light, there are *alternate dark and light bands of varying widths originating at dentinoenamel junction* and *running outwards* and ending at some distance from the outer surface of enamel (Fig. 2.8). These are called as *Hunter—Schreger bands*. The *dark bands* are called *diazones* and *light bands* are called *parazones*. It has been suggested that presence or appearance of these bands correspond with *variation in calcification of enamel*. However, it has been widely accepted that it is an optical phenomenon as a result of change in the direction of enamel rods.

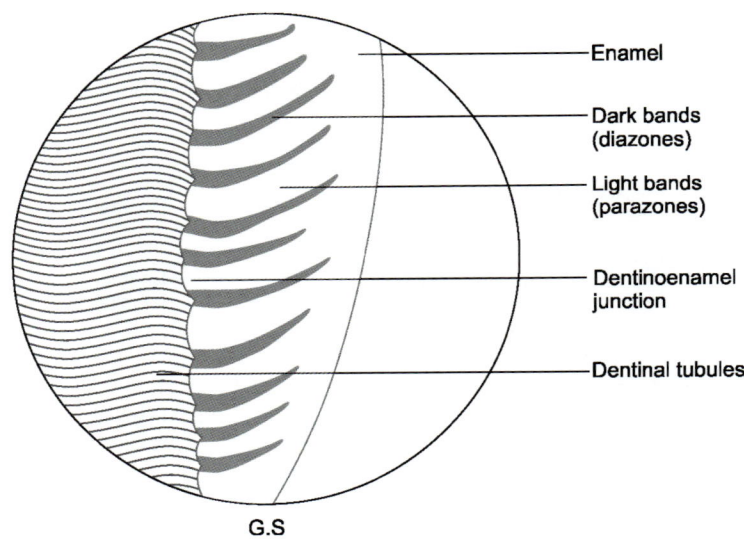

Figure 2.8   Hunter–Schreger bands — alternate light and dark bands originating at dentinoenamel junction and running outward.

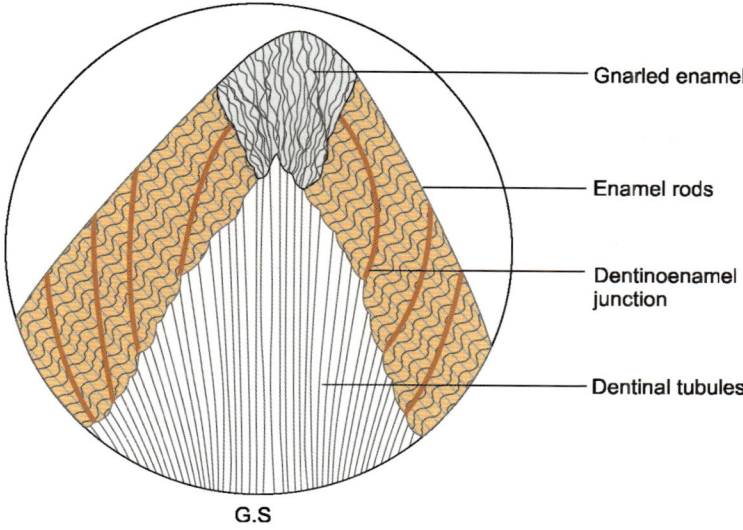

Gnarled enamel

Enamel rods

Dentinoenamel
junction

Dentinal tubules

G.S

Figure 2.9   Gnarled enamel — complex arrangement of enamel rods.

GNARLED ENAMEL

Usually the enamel rods are perpendicular to the dentinoenamel junction. However, in some areas, especially *in the region of cusps*, the *rods* appear to be *twisted around each other* and thus, making *more complex arrangement of rods*. Such areas are called as gnarled enamel (Fig. 2.9).It may be considered as an *optical phenomenon* and supposed to be *associated with increased strength of enamel.*

Dentin 3

DENTINAL TUBULES

Histologically, dentin is characterized by the presence of *closely packed dentinal tubules and dentin matrix* (Fig. 3.1A and B). These dentinal tubules contain *cytoplasmic processes of odontoblasts* which are arranged in a layer along the peripheral boundary of the dental pulp. These tubules *run from the pulpal surface towards the dentinoenamel junction* in crown *and dentinocemental junction* in root and end *perpendicular to these junctions*. These are about 3−4 microns in diameter near the pulpal cavity and about 1 micron at their outer ends. They follow a gentle *S-shaped course* (curved, sigmoid course) which is more pronounced in the crown and less in the root. They are perpendicular to the pulpal surface, with the *first convexity* of this S-shaped curvature directed *towards the apex of the root*. This is known as *primary curve*. These tubules are almost straight along the incisal edges, cusps and near root tip. The tubules show *relatively minute curvatures* throughout their entire length which are known as *secondary curvatures*. These tubules show *branching near the dentinoenamel junction* and are known as *terminal branches*. These dentinal tubules have *lateral branches* which are somewhat at right angle to the main dentinal tubule, 1 micron or less in diameter and about every 1−2 microns along the length and are termed as *canaliculi or microtubules*.

INCREMENTAL LINES

Incremental lines of von Ebner in dentin are similar to incremental lines in enamel (Fig. 3.2). They appear as fine lines or striations in dentin and indicate the *daily rhythmic, recurrent deposition of dentin matrix* as well as a *hesitation in a daily formative process*. The distance between these lines vary

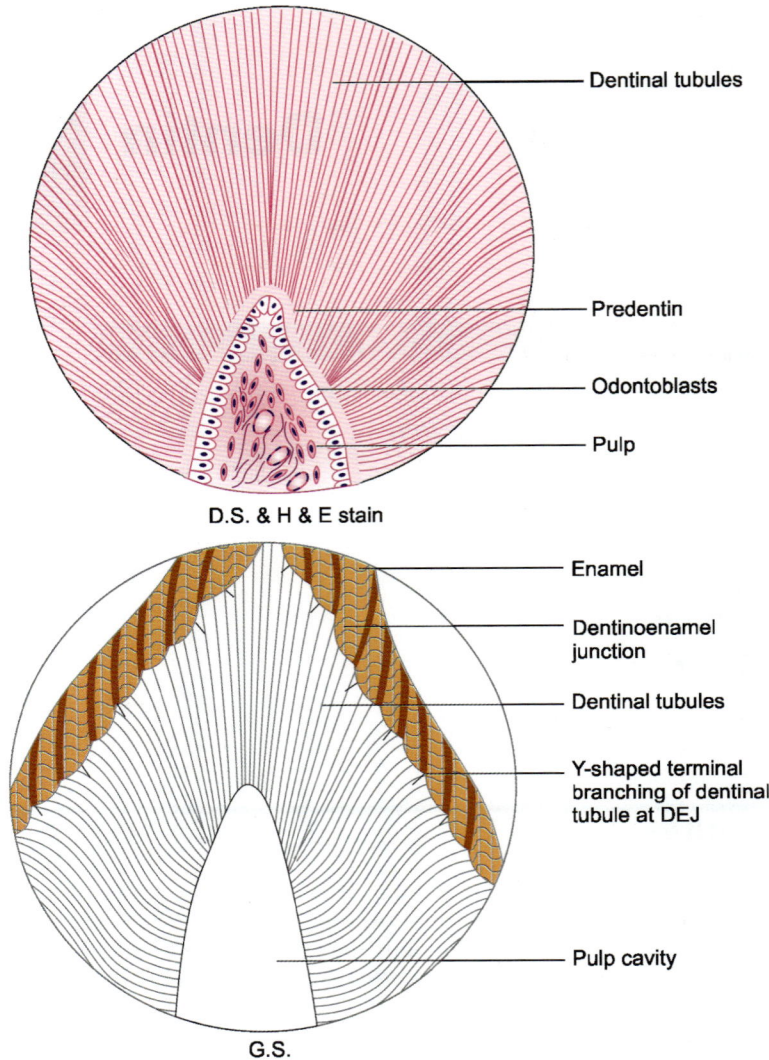

D.S. & H & E stain

— Dentinal tubules

— Predentin

— Odontoblasts

— Pulp

— Enamel

— Dentinoenamel junction

— Dentinal tubules

— Y-shaped terminal branching of dentinal tubule at DEJ

— Pulp cavity

G.S.

Figure 3.1 (A) Dentinal tubules – dentin characterized by presence of closely packed dentinal tubules. (B) Dentinal tubules – dentinal tubules with S-shaped curvature and Y-shaped terminal branching at dentinoenamel junction.

from 4 to 8 microns in crown and less in root. They run at *right angles to the dentinal tubules* and the *course of these lines* indicates the *growth pattern of the dentin.*

Some of these *incremental lines are accentuated* due *to disturbances in the matrix and mineralization process.* These lines are called as *contour lines of Owen.* However, some investigators are of the opinion that these lines are due to coincidence of secondary curvatures between neighbouring dentinal tubules. Inadequate nutrition and periods of illness are also indicated by accentuated contour lines within the dentin.

The dentin is formed partly before birth and partly after birth in deciduous teeth and first permanent molars. This *prenatal and postnatal dentin* is separated by an *accentuated contour line* which is known as *neonatal line.* This line indicates abrupt change in the environment which occurs at birth and may be a *hypocalcified structure* in dentin. *Prenatal dentin* is usually of *better quality* than postnatal dentin.

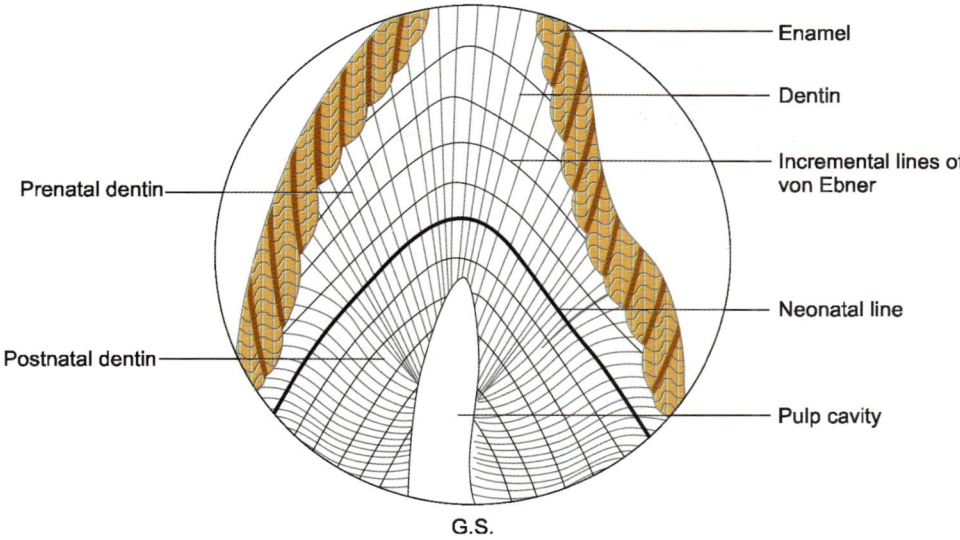

Figure 3.2 Incremental lines – incremental lines of von Ebner as fine lines in dentin and neonatal line separating prenatal and postnatal dentin.

INTERGLOBULAR DENTIN

Mineralization of dentin takes place *as globules or calcospherites* which usually fuse to form a uniformly calcified tissue. However, in some areas, these *globules fail to fuse* (fusion is incomplete) and this results in *zones of hypomineralization* between the globules. These zones are known as *globular dentin or interglobular spaces* (Fig. 3.3). These are prominently *seen in crowns of teeth* in the circumpulpal dentin *just below the mantle dentin*. Dentinal tubules pass through these areas without any deviation thus indicating that it is a defect of mineralization and not of matrix formation. In ground sections, these areas appear *dark (black) in transmitted light* due to internal reflection of light.

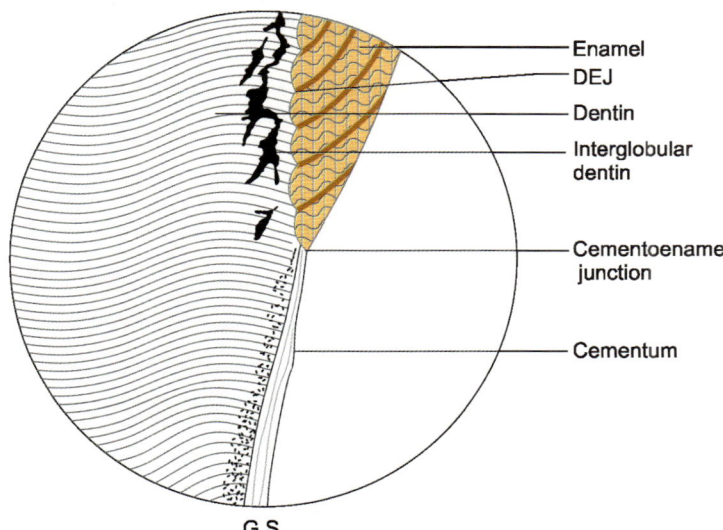

Figure 3.3 Interglobular dentin — interglobular dentin appearing dark below the dentinoenamel junction.

TOMES' GRANULAR LAYER

In ground section, under transmitted light, a *granular appearing area* is seen *in the root dentin adjacent to cementum*. This is known as *Tomes' granular layer* (Fig. 3.4). There is a progressive increase in amount of this layer from cementoenamel junction to the root apex. These are supposed to be the *result of coalescing and looping of terminal portions of the dentinal tubules*. Alternatively, it has been suggested that it may be due to the incomplete fusion of calcospherites.

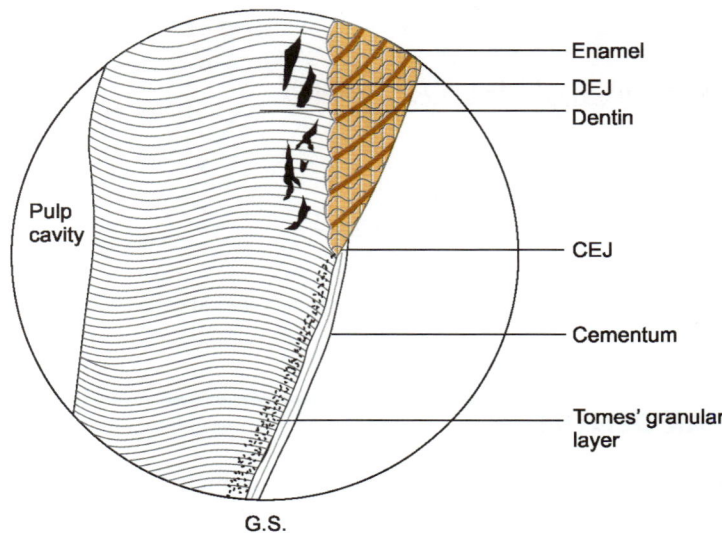

Figure 3.4 Tomes' granular layer – Tomes' granular layer appearing as a granular area in the root dentin adjacent to cementum.

PERITUBULAR AND INTERTUBULAR DENTIN

The dentin which is *present around the odontoblastic process and forms the wall of the dentinal tubule* is known as peritubular dentin. It is *also known as intratubular dentin* (Fig. 3.5). *Dentin located between the dentinal tubules* is *known as intertubular dentin.*

The *peritubular dentin* is *more highly calcified* than intertubular dentin. It consists of inorganic apatite crystals with small amount of organic matrix. In *decalcified section* under light microscopy, the *peritubular dentin appears as an empty space surrounding the odontoblastic process.*

The *intertubular dentin forms* the *main body of the dentin* and is *present between the zones of peritubular dentin.* It is the primary secretory product of odontoblast. It is retained after decalcification, though it is highly mineralized. It consists of collagenous material, organic ground substance and smaller amount of apatite crystals.

PRIMARY AND SECONDARY DENTIN

The dentin which is *formed before root completion* is known as *primary dentin* (Fig. 3.6). It *consists of mantle dentin and circumpulpal dentin. Mantle dentin* is the *first formed dentin* in the crown and is present *just below the dentinoenamel junction. Circumpulpal dentin* forms *the remaining part of the*

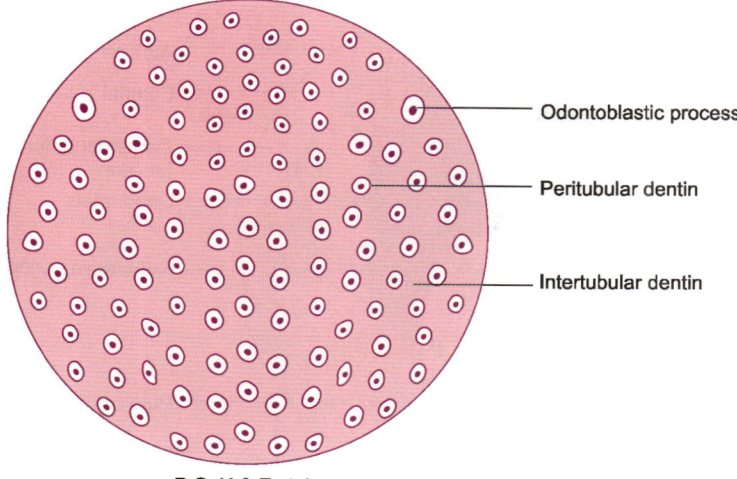

D.S. H & E stain

Figure 3.5 Peritubular and intertubular dentin – the dentin present around the odontoblastic process and forming the wall of the dentinal tubule is peritubular dentin appearing as an empty space surrounding the odontoblastic process in D.S. The dentin present in between the zones of peritubular dentin is the intertubular dentin.

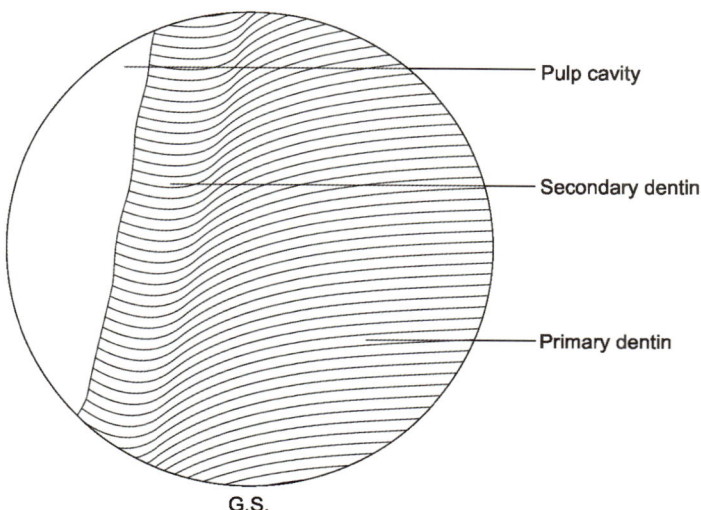

G.S.

Figure 3.6 Primary and secondary dentin – dentinal tubules bend as they pass from primary into secondary dentin. Secondary dentin is a narrow band of dentin bordering the pulp.

primary dentin or bulk of the tooth. It is *present between mantle dentin and predentin.* The circumpulpal dentin is slightly more mineralized than the mantle dentin.

The *dentin which is formed after root completion* is known as *secondary dentin* (Fig. 3.6). It is *a narrow band of dentin bordering pulp.* There is a bend in the tubules where primary and secondary dentin interface. The structure of secondary dentin is similar to primary dentin. It has been proposed that the rate of deposition of secondary dentin by odontoblast is slow and contains few tubules. It is formed in greater amounts on the roof and floor of the coronal pulp chamber and thus *protects the pulp.*

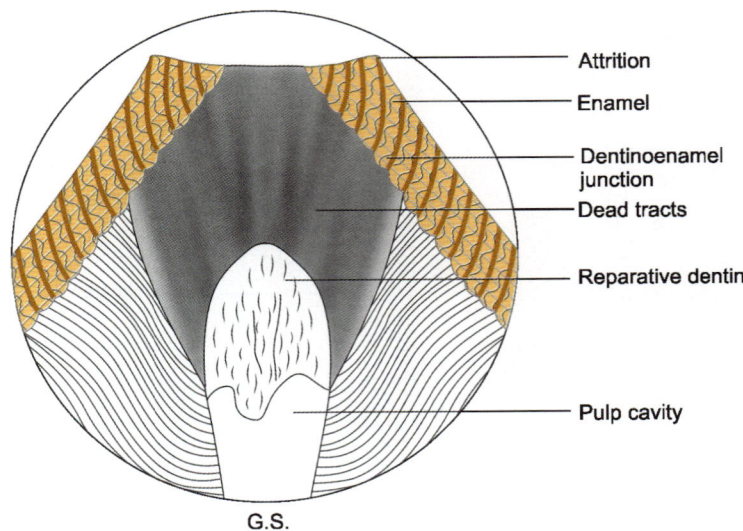

G.S.

Figure 3.7 Dead tracts and reparative dentin – flattening of occlusal surface with formation of dead tracts and reparative dentin.

DEAD TRACTS AND REPARATIVE DENTIN

Dead tracts are the *areas in dentin* characterized by *degenerated odontoblast processes* (Fig. 3.7). In dried ground sections of tooth, the odontoblast processes disintegrate and the empty dentinal tubules are filled with air. These air-filled tubules *appear black in transmitted light and white in reflected light.* Loss of odontoblastic processes *may also occur due to caries, attrition, abrasion, erosion or cavity preparation* in the teeth with vital pulp.

Reparative dentin (tertiary dentin or reactive dentin) is formed *as a response to various stimuli* such as attrition, abrasion, erosion, carious or operative procedures (Fig. 3.7). Due to these stimuli, the odontoblastic processes are exposed or cut and the odontoblasts also die or survive. If the odontoblasts survive, the dentin produced is known as reactionary dentin. If the odontoblasts die, they are replaced by the new odontoblasts from the cells of the pulp (either from cells in cell rich zone or undifferentiated perivascular cells). These newly differentiated odontoblasts form a dentin known as reparative dentin. The formation of reparative dentin *acts as a healing process.* It has *few tubules and twisted course* of the tubules than normal dentin. Sometimes *dentin-forming cells get included in rapidly forming matrix;* this is called as *osteodentin.*

SCLEROTIC OR TRANSPARENT DENTIN

Sclerotic dentin are the *areas where dentinal tubules are obliterated with calcified material* (Fig. 3.8). These are the *hypercalcified areas.* It is seen in the *teeth of older individuals,* especially in *root dentin.* The lumen of the dentinal tubule is obliterated with calcified material and the refractive indices of dentin in which the tubules are occluded are same and these areas appear transparent. It appears *transparent (light) in transmitted light and dark in reflected light.* It may also be formed as a result of caries, attrition, abrasion, erosion or cavity preparation as a *protective phenomenon.* It reduces the permeability of dentin and prolongs the vitality of pulp. It was found to be harder than normal dentin.

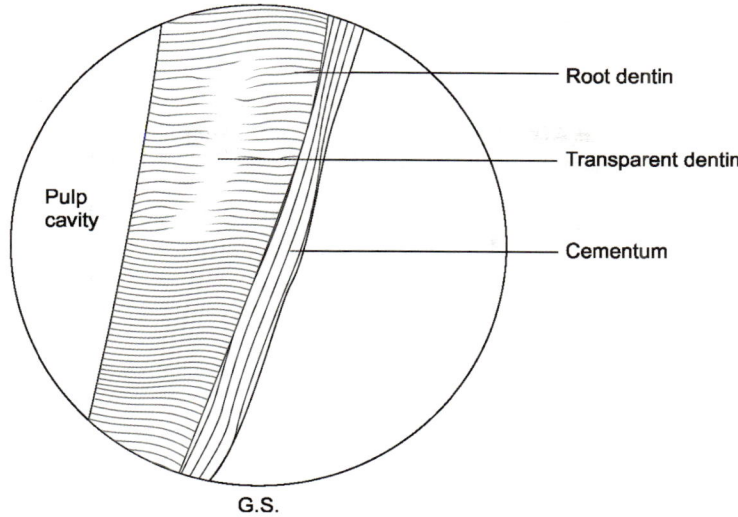

G.S.

Figure 3.8 Sclerotic or transparent dentin – transparent dentin appearing light.

PREDENTIN

The *dentin* is initially laid down as a *layer of unmineralized matrix* called *predentin* (Fig. 3.9). It is always located adjacent to pulp tissue. It consists of collagen fibres and amorphous ground substance. As the collagen fibres undergo mineralization at the predentin−dentin junction, this predentin becomes dentin and a new layer of predentin is formed by odontoblasts circumpulpally. The *width of predentin* varies from *2 to 6 microns* depending on activity of odontoblasts. The rate of formation of predentin diminishes with age. In decalcified and haematoxylin and

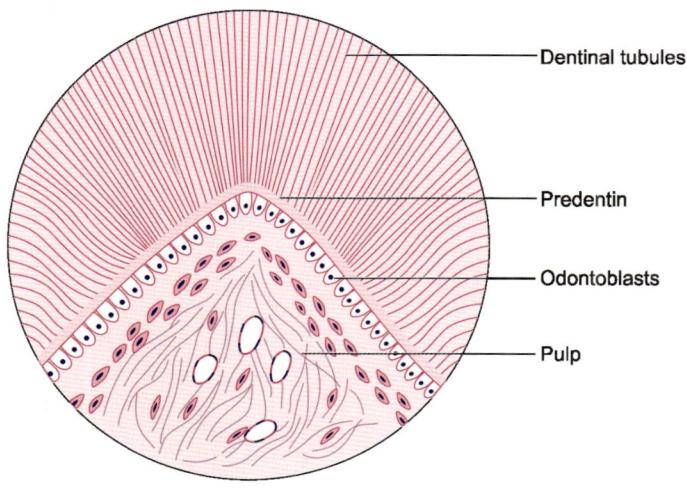

D.S. H & E stain

Figure 3.9 Predentin – predentin appearing as a pale staining area which is an unmineralized matrix adjacent to the pulp tissue.

eosin–stained sections of tooth, it appears as a *pale staining (staining less intensely)* than mineralized dentin.

Transmitted light: The light that has passed through a transparent medium. The light is transmitted from a source on the opposite side of the specimen to the objective lens. Usually, the light is passed through the condenser to focus it on the specimen to get the maximum illumination.

Reflected light: The light rays are thrown back by illuminated object such as mirror.

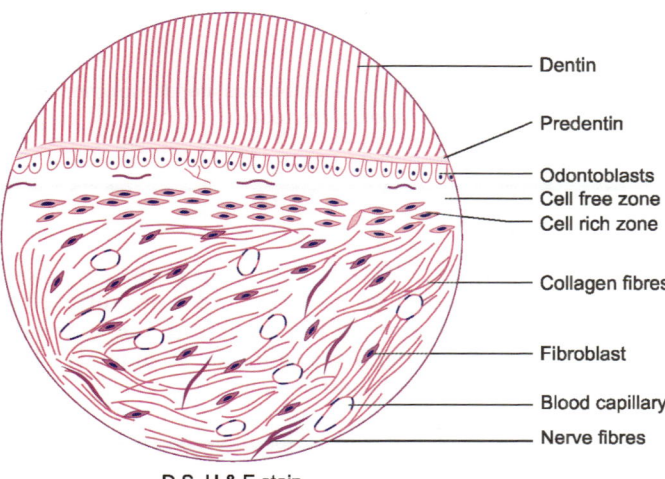

Pulp 4

PULP AT PERIPHERY

Dental pulp is a loose connective tissue and consists of cells and intercellular substance. Peripherally, the pulp (Fig. 4.1) is composed of:

i. *Odontoblasts* which are formative cells of dentin.
ii. *Cell-free zone or zone of Weil* which is beneath the odontoblasts and is a space in which the odontoblasts may move towards the pulp during tooth development. It is prominent in coronal pulp.

D.S. H & E stain

Figure 4.1 Pulp at periphery – pulp at periphery shows odontoblasts, cell-free zone, cell-rich zone and pulp core.

iii. *Cell-rich zone* which is adjacent to cell-free zone and cell density is high and composed mainly of *fibroblasts and undifferentiated mesenchymal cells* and is easily seen in coronal pulp.

iv. *Pulp core* which shows presence of major vessels and nerves of the pulp.

ODONTOBLASTS AT DIFFERENT LEVELS IN THE PULP

Odontoblasts, the formative cells of dentin are present in the pulp adjacent to predentin with *cell bodies in the pulp and cell processes* extending *into predentin and dentin* within the dentinal tubules (Fig. 4.2). They form a single layer of cells. The number of odontoblasts is similar to the number of dentinal tubules. The *shape of odontoblasts* varies in different regions of the tooth. They are more *cylindrical and tall columnar in the crown,* more *cuboidal* in the *middle of the root and ovoid or spindle shaped* close to the *apex of the tooth.*

The cell bodies of odontoblasts are columnar in shape with large nuclei in the basal (pulpal) region of the cell. In light microscope, an active cell appears elongated with basophilic cytoplasm and basally placed nucleus. A resting cell is with little cytoplasm and more haematoxyphilic nucleus.

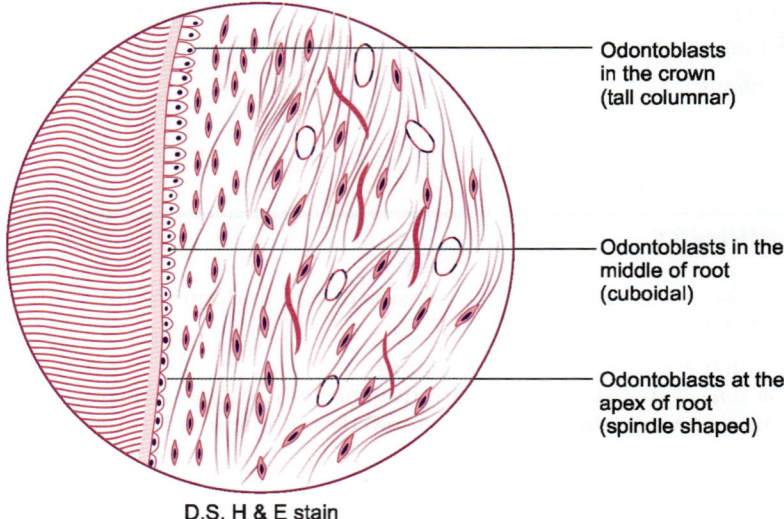

Odontoblasts in the crown (tall columnar)

Odontoblasts in the middle of root (cuboidal)

Odontoblasts at the apex of root (spindle shaped)

D.S. H & E stain

Figure 4.2   Odontoblasts at different levels in the pulp – odontoblasts are tall, columnar in the crown, cuboidal in the middle of the root and spindle shaped close to the apex of the tooth.

PULP FIBROSIS

Pulp fibrosis is a *regressive change* in aging pulp (Fig. 4.3). Pulp shows *deposition of bundles of collagen fibres and diffused fibrillar components.* The fibres are arranged more diffusely in coronal pulp and longitudinally in radicular pulp. It is a gradual phenomenon and may occur *as a result of any external trauma* such as dental caries or deep restorations. It may also be due to increase in collagen in medial and adventitial layers of blood vessels.

PULP STONES (TRUE)

Pulp stones are *nodular, mineralized structures* seen in coronal and/or radicular pulp tissue (Fig. 4.4A).

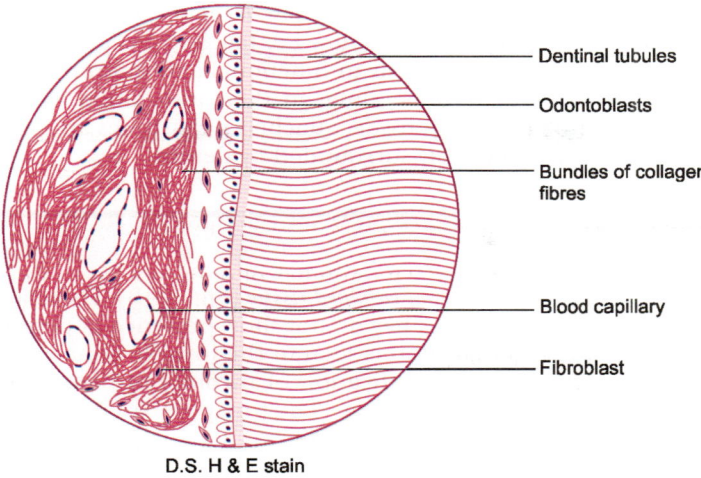

Dentinal tubules

Odontoblasts

Bundles of collagen fibres

Blood capillary

Fibroblast

D.S. H & E stain

Figure 4.3 Pulp fibrosis – deposition of dense collagen fibre bundles.

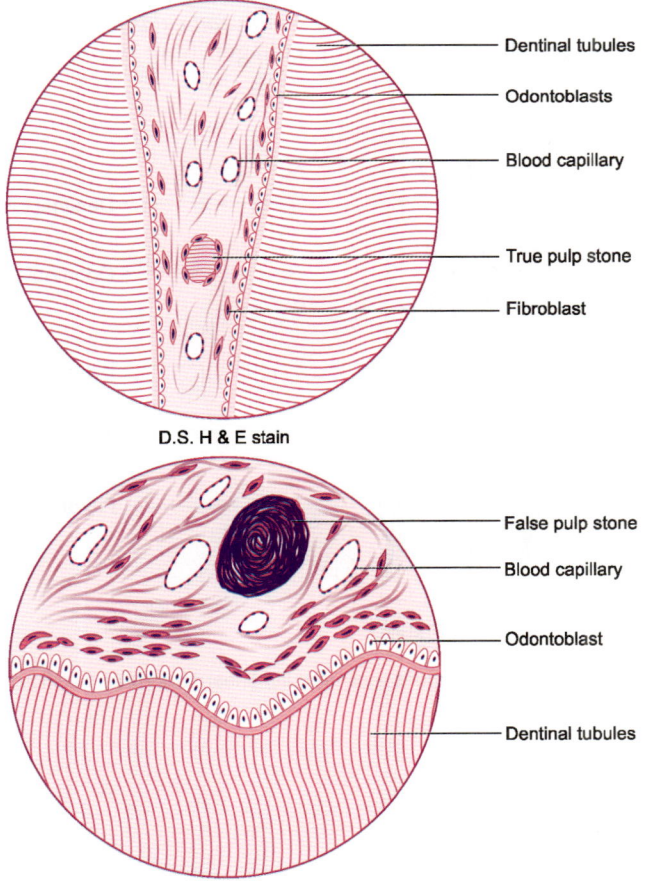

Dentinal tubules

Odontoblasts

Blood capillary

True pulp stone

Fibroblast

D.S. H & E stain

False pulp stone

Blood capillary

Odontoblast

Dentinal tubules

D.S. H & E stain

Figure 4.4 (A) Pulp stones (true) – true pulp stone which resembles the dentin and odontoblasts are seen on the surface. (B) Pulp stones (false) – false pulp stone as concentric layers of calcified tissue.

True pulp stones are rare and commonly seen *close to apical foramen*. These are formed by *odontoblasts* and *resemble secondary dentin in structure*, i.e. few and irregular dentinal tubules and odontoblasts on their surface. They may occur in functional and unerupted teeth. They may be subdivided as *free, attached or embedded* depending on their association with dentin. Free pulp stones are completely surrounded by pulp tissue, attached pulp stones are partly fused to dentin and embedded pulp stones are completely surrounded by dentin.

PULP STONES (FALSE)

False pulp stones appear as *concentric layers of calcified tissue* (Fig. 4.4B). These are more *common in pulp chambers* as compared to root canals. They do not show presence of dentinal tubules. There is a central nidus around which calcification is seen in the form of concentric layers. It may be remnants of necrotic or calcified cells, calcification of thrombi of blood vessels (phleboliths) or calcification within a collagen fibre bundle. They may be subdivided as *free, attached or embedded* depending on their association with dentin.

DIFFUSE CALCIFICATIONS

Diffuse calcifications are *amorphous dystrophic calcifications* which appear as *irregular linear strands of calcific deposits* (Fig. 4.5). They are most *commonly seen in radicular pulp* and supposed to be an age related degenerative change. They usually follow collagen fibre bundles or blood vessels.

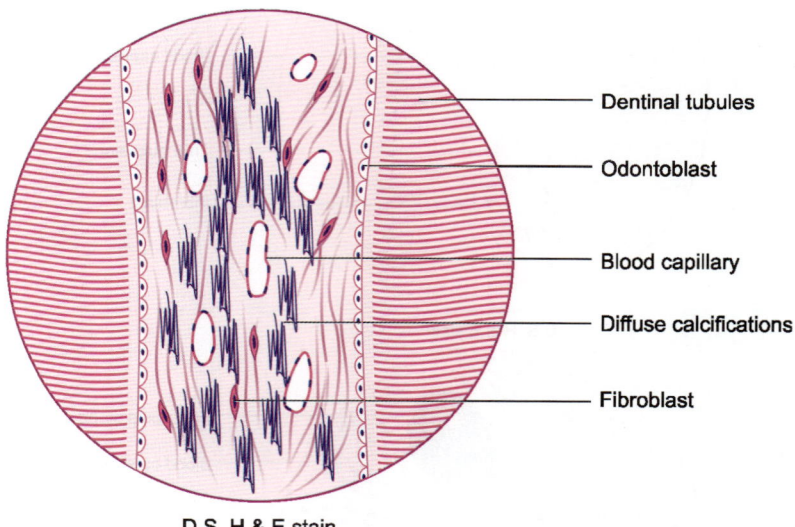

Dentinal tubules

Odontoblast

Blood capillary

Diffuse calcifications

Fibroblast

D.S. H & E stain

Figure 4.5   Diffuse calcifications – as irregular linear strands of calcific deposits.

Cementum 5

ACELLULAR CEMENTUM

Acellular cementum is also known as *primary cementum* (first formed layer). It *extends from cementoe-namel junction to the apex of the root* (Fig. 5.1). However, it is *usually present in the cervical third of the root*. The *rate of matrix formation* is relatively *slow* in acellular cementum than cellular cementum. *Embedded cementocytes* are absent in acellular cementum. *Incremental lines* of acellular cementum tend to be *close together, thin and regular*.

The *periodontal ligament fibres* that *enter the cementum* are termed as *Sharpey's fibres* which run perpendicular to the surface of the cementum.

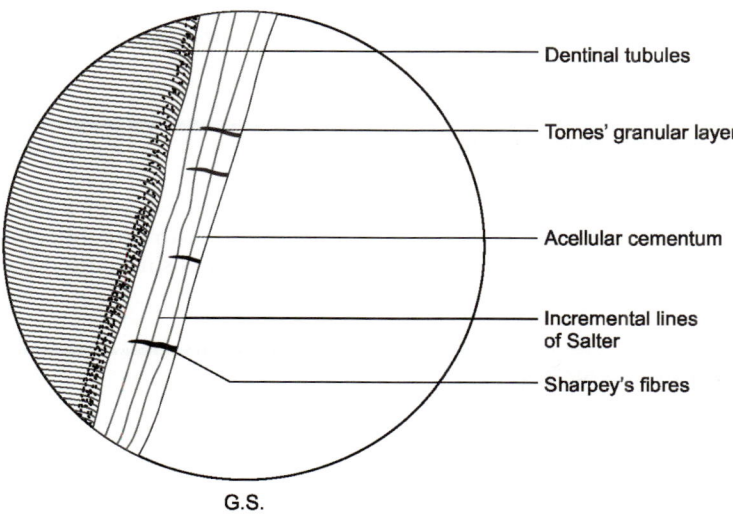

Dentinal tubules

Tomes' granular layer

Acellular cementum

Incremental lines of Salter

Sharpey's fibres

G.S.

Figure 5.1 Acellular cementum – acellular cementum and Sharpey's fibres.

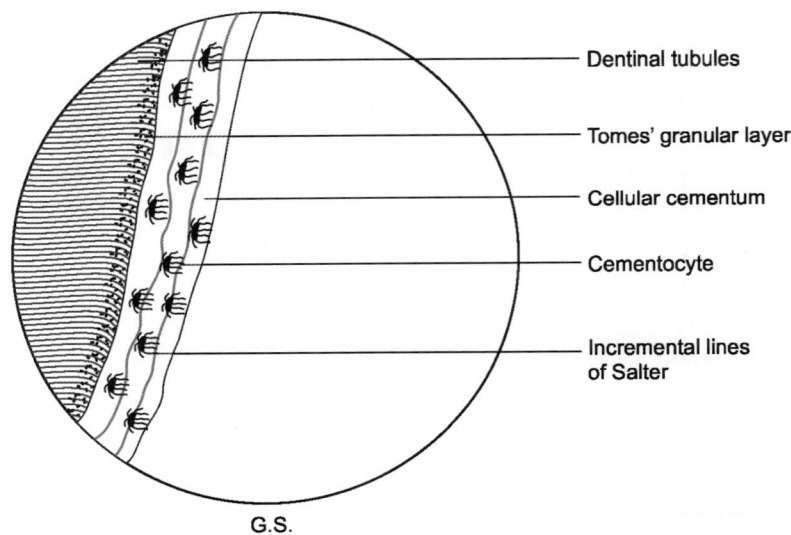

Dentinal tubules

Tomes' granular layer

Cellular cementum

Cementocyte

Incremental lines of Salter

G.S.

Figure 5.2 Cellular cementum – cellular cementum with cementocytes in lacunae with cell processes in canaliculi, most of which canaliculi are directed towards the external surface, i.e. periodontal ligament.

CELLULAR CEMENTUM

Cellular cementum is also known as *secondary cementum* (Fig. 5.2). It is formed after the formation of acellular cementum. It is *mainly present at the apical third and interradicular area*. The *rate of deposition is faster. Embedded cementocytes are present* in cellular cementum. These *cementocytes* are entrapped cementoblasts which lie *in spaces* called *lacunae* and their *processes* lie in *canaliculi*. Most of these *canaliculi* are oriented *towards the periodontal ligament* being the chief source of nutrition. These are more widely dispersed and more randomly arranged as compared to osteocytes in bone. In ground sections, the cellular contents are lost and the voids get filled with air and debris due to which they appear dark. In decalcified sections, the cellular contents of the lacunae are retained and cementocytes appear as shrunken cells. *Incremental lines* in cellular cementum tend to be *wide apart, thicker and more irregular.*

INCREMENTAL LINES OF SALTER

Incremental lines of Salter represent the *periods of rest during cementum formation* (Fig. 5.3). These lines run *parallel to the long axis of the root*. These are *highly mineralized* with less collagen fibres and more ground substance. They can be best seen in haematoxylin and eosin–stained decalcified sections as haematoxyphilic lines.

CEMENTOENAMEL JUNCTION

It is the *relation between cementum and enamel at the cervical region* which is variable (Fig. 5.4). In approximately *60%* of teeth, *cementum overlaps the cervical end of enamel* for a short distance. It is due to degeneration of enamel epithelium at the cervical end which permits the direct contact of connective tissue with the enamel surface. The cementum thus produced is afibrillar cementum.

In approximately *30%* of teeth, *cementum and enamel meet* in *relatively sharp line* at the cervical end of enamel.

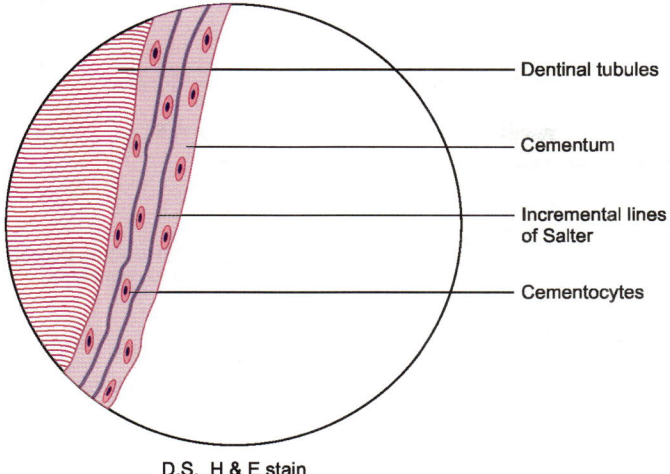

D.S. H & E stain

Figure 5.3 Incremental lines of Salter – incremental lines of Salter as haematoxyphilic lines which indicate periods of rest during cementum formation.

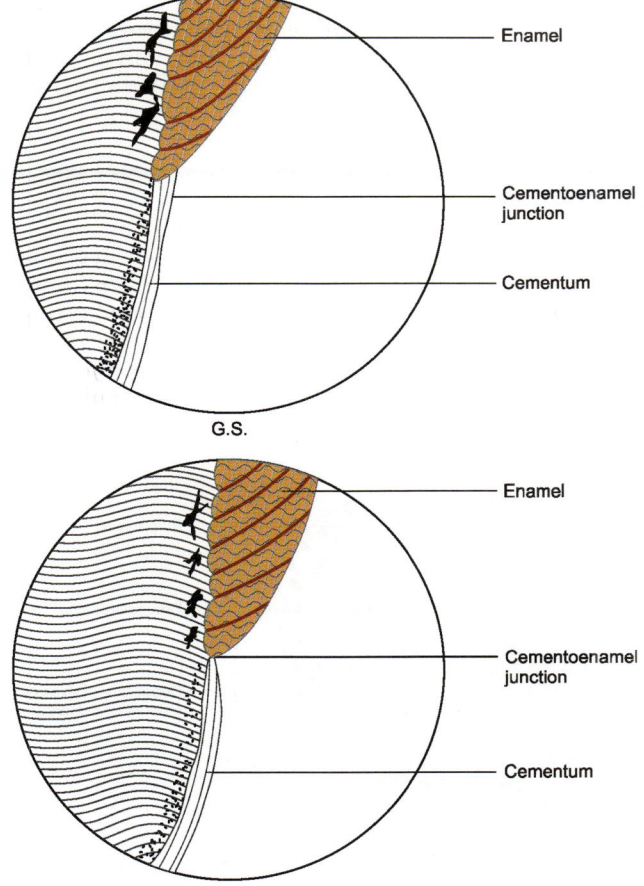

Figure 5.4 Cementoenamel junction: (A) overlap – CEJ where cementum overlaps the cervical end of enamel for a short distance, (B) at a sharp point – CEJ where cementum and enamel meet at a sharp line at the cervical end of enamel and

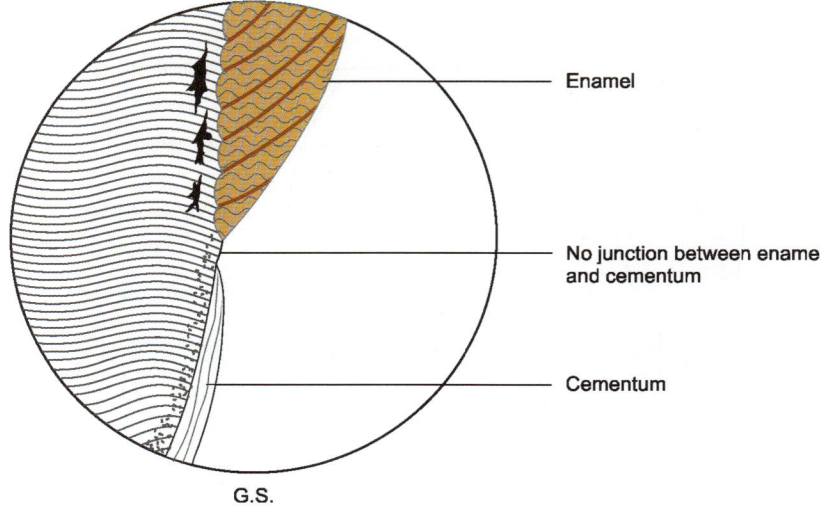

G.S.

Figure 5.4, cont'd   (C) no junction – where cementum and enamel do not meet, there is a gap between cementum and enamel.

In approximately *10%* of teeth, *cementum and enamel do not meet*. In such cases, there is no cementoenamel junction and there is a gap between cementum and enamel, exposing root dentin. It may occur when there is a delay in separation of enamel epithelium from dentin in the cervical portion of the root.

HYPERCEMENTOSIS

Hypercementosis is an *abnormal thickening of cementum* (Fig. 5.5). It may affect all the teeth of the dentition or a single tooth or only parts of a tooth. It may be *circumscribed or diffuse* (localized or generalized). It occurs *physiologically due to accelerated eruption of teeth. Localized hypertrophy* as a spur or prong-like extensions of cementum is seen *in teeth* which are *exposed to great stress. Circumscribed extensive deposition* of cementum is associated with *chronic periapical infections. Generalized hypercementosis* is seen in *Paget disease.* Localized thickening may be seen in benign cementoblastoma, florid cemento-osseous dysplasia, acromegaly and calcinosis.

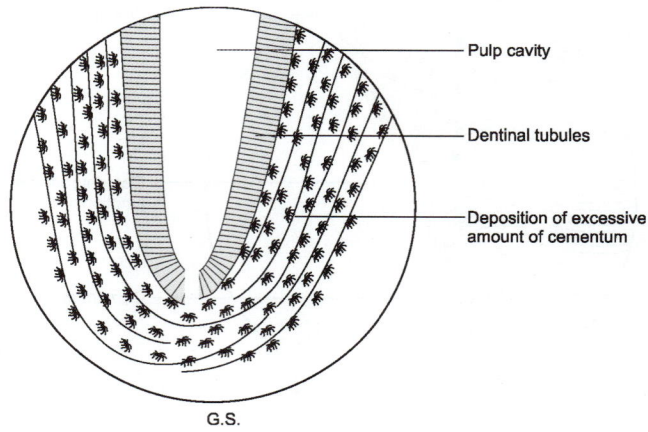

G.S.

Figure 5.5   Hypercementosis – deposition of excessive amount of cementum.

Periodontal Ligament 6

PRINCIPAL FIBRES

The majority of connective tissue fibres of periodontal ligament are *collagen fibres*. These collagen fibre bundles, arranged in groups, are the principal fibres of periodontal ligament which *extends from cementum to the alveolus* (Fig. 6.1). It has been suggested that these fibres do not *run a* straight course, instead they run in a *wavy course*.

These are arranged in *five groups*:

i) Alveolar crest group: These fibres *extend from cervical cementum to alveolar crest* and to the fibrous layer of periosteum covering the alveolar bone.

ii) Horizontal group: These fibres *extend from cementum to alveolar bone* and are *at right angles to the long axis of the tooth*. These are found just apical to the alveolar crest group.

iii) Oblique group: These fibres are the *most numerous* and extend *from cementum to the alveolar bone in oblique direction with coronal position* into the *alveolar bone* and *apical position* into the *cementum*.

iv) Apical group: These fibres *extend from cementum around the apex of the root* to the bone *at the base of the socket*.

v) Interradicular group: These fibres are found in *multirooted teeth* and extend *from cementum into the bone forming the crest of interradicular septum*.

EPITHELIAL RESTS OF MALASSEZ

Epithelial rests of Malassez, first described by *Malassez* are the *remnants of Hertwig's epithelial root sheath* (Fig. 6.2) and found in *periodontal ligament close to the cementum surface* (about 25 microns from the cementum surface). During the cementum formation, the continuous layer of epithelium covering the surface of newly formed dentin breaks into lace like strands. These epithelial rests *persist as a network, islands, strands or tubule-like structures* near and *parallel to the root surface* in tangential or serial sections. They appear as cluster-like in cross-section. These are separated from the surrounding connective tissue by a basal lamina. In *H&E-stained section*, they appear as *closely packed cuboidal cells with a deeply stained nucleus*. Their distribution varies according to age and site.

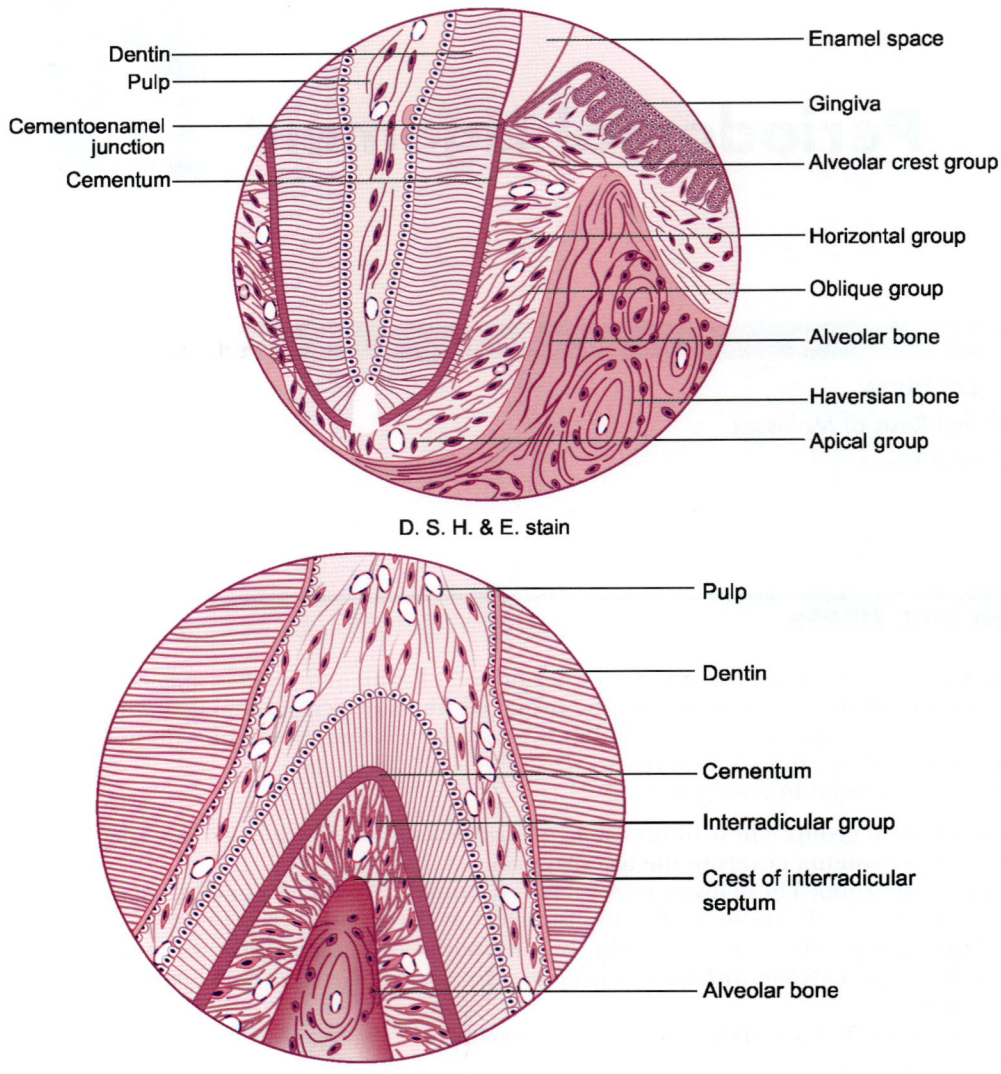

Figure 6.1   (A) Principal fibres – arrangement of principal fibre group of periodontal ligament. (B) Interradicular group of principal fibres – interradicular group of fibres seen in multirooted teeth.

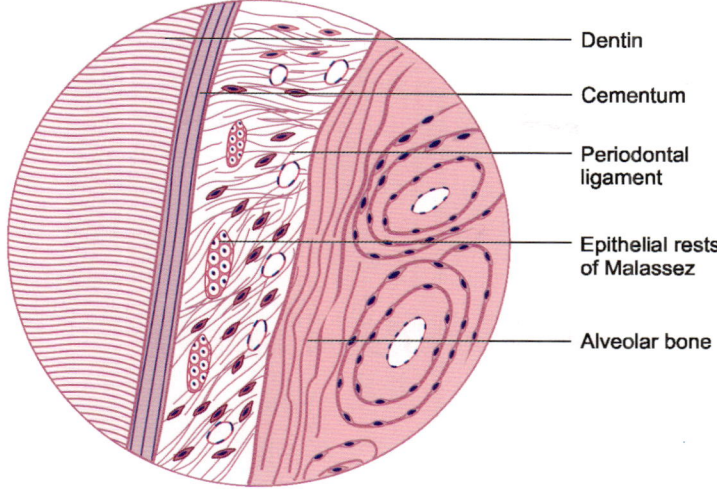

D. S. H. & E. stain

Figure 6.2 Epithelial rests of Malassez – epithelial rests of Malassez present in periodontal ligament close to the cementum surface as islands appearing as closely packed cuboidal cells with deeply staining nucleus.

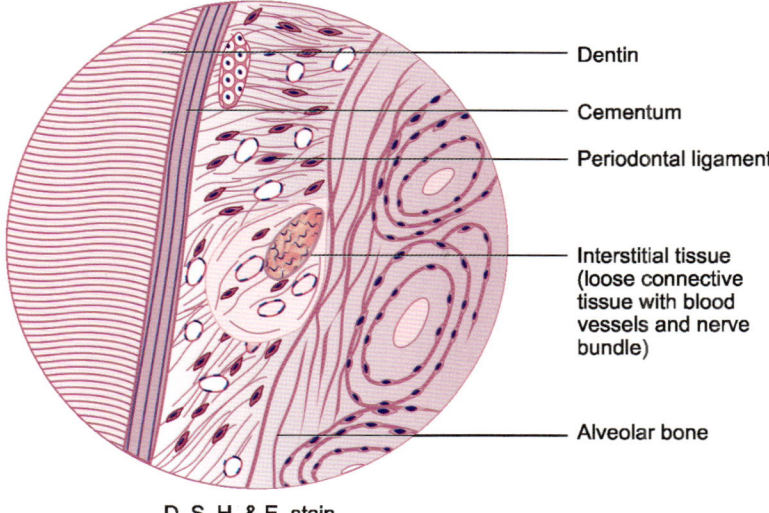

D. S. H. & E. stain

Figure 6.3 Interstitial tissue – loose connective tissue in periodontal ligament with blood vessels and nerve bundle.

These are more numerous in children and less numerous in older individuals. These are more in number in the furcation area. These cells *may undergo proliferation to form cysts and tumours* or may undergo calcification to *form cementicles.*

INTERSTITIAL TISSUE

Interstitial tissue is a *loose connective tissue* in which *blood vessels, nerves and lymphatics* of the *periodontal ligament* are present (Fig. 6.3). The collagen fibres are less regularly arranged.

Alveolar Bone 7

OSTEOBLASTS AND OSTEOCYTES

Osteoblasts are specialized cells of mesenchymal origin *arising from pluripotent stem cells* (Fig. 7.1). These are the *formative cells of bone* and are seen prominently as a cell layer over the forming bone. *Active osteoblasts* appear as *plump cuboidal cells with round nucleus* and *basophilic cytoplasm* due to abundant endoplasmic reticulum within the cells. These osteoblasts secrete an *unmineralized layer* known as *osteoid* which is the organic matrix and made up of collagen and the noncollagenous proteins. *High alkaline phosphatase activity* is seen in *osteoblasts*. They appear as flattened cells when there is no bone formation.

When the *osteoblasts* form the bone matrix, some of them get *entrapped within the matrix*, these cells are *called osteocytes* (Fig. 7.1). Within the bone matrix, osteocytes get reduced in size. These are present within the bone. The number of osteocytes depends on the rate of bone formation, rapid the rate of bone formation, more osteocytes are seen per unit volume. Osteocytes are lost during preparation of ground section, the spaces or lacunae in which they are present get filled with the cell debris or air and they appear back in transmitted light under light microscopy. *Numerous cell processes* of the osteocytes are present in the *canaliculi* which run in *all directions*. These *osteocytes* are more *regularly distributed than the cementocytes* in the cementum. In decalcified section, osteocytes are retained but canaliculi are not seen.

OSTEOCLASTS

Osteoclasts are the *large multinucleated physiologic giant cells* responsible for *resorption of bone*, derived from haemopoietic cells of monocytes – microphage lineage (Fig. 7.2). They are *found* along the resorbing surfaces of bone in *resorption concavities* called as *Howship's lacunae*. They show variation in size and shape due to their motility. Usually these are *larger cells*

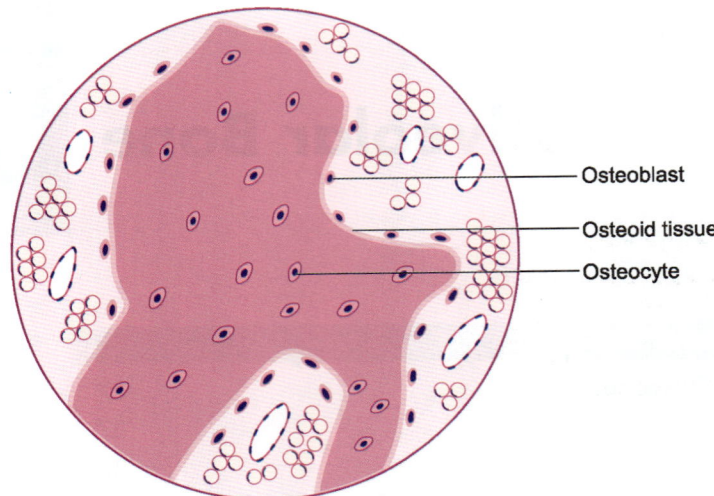

Figure 7.1   Osteoblasts and osteocytes – active osteoblasts appear as cuboidal cells with basophilic cytoplasm and round nucleus. There is pale staining osteoid tissue suggestive of bone formation. Osteocytes are seen within the bone.

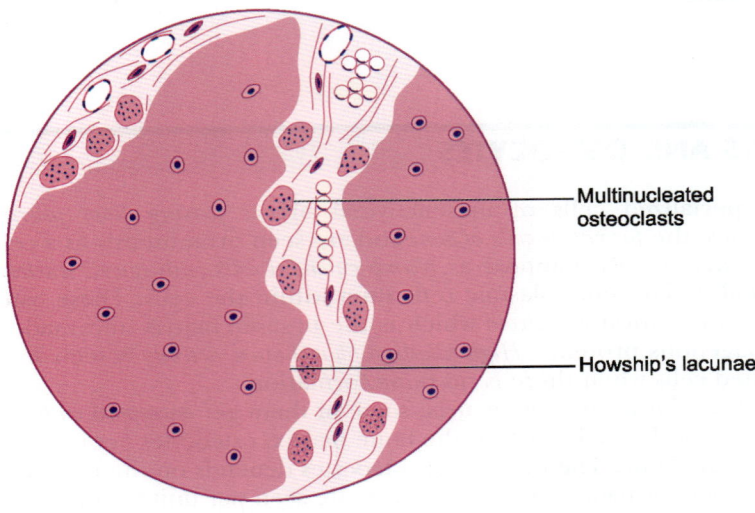

D.S. H & E stain

Figure 7.2   Osteoclasts – large multinucleated giant cells in Howship's lacunae.

approximately 40–100 microns in diameter with an average *10–20 closely packed nuclei.* The *cell membrane* adjacent to bone where resorption takes place has a *striated appearance* (deep infoldings of cell membranes) and this is the *ruffled border* of osteoclasts. The acid phosphatase activity differentiates the osteoclast from other multinucleated giant cells.

COMPACT BONE

Compact bone, also *called lamellar bone,* shows *dense bone mass arranged in layers* with more regular distribution of osteocytes (Fig. 7.3). Ground section of compact bone shows

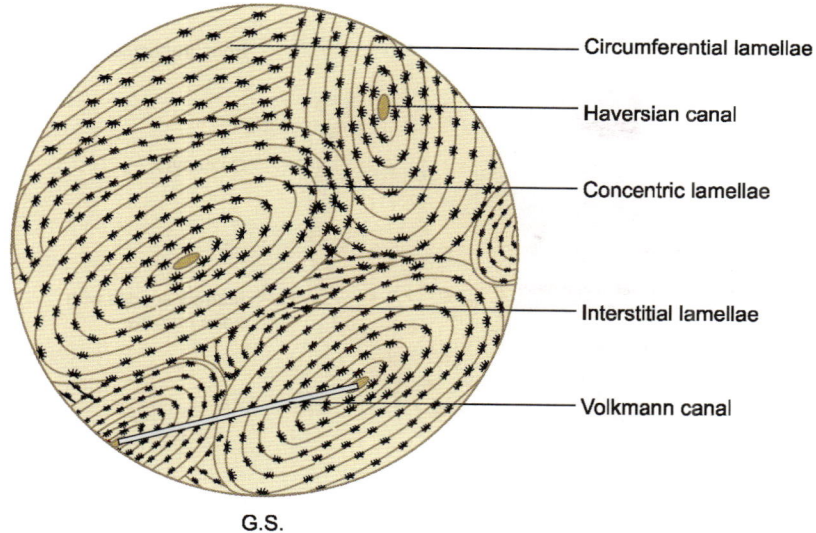

G.S.

Figure 7.3 Compact bone – compact bone consists of Haversian system or osteon. In the centre of each osteon, there is a Haversian canal around which concentric lamellae are arranged. Interstitial lamellae are present between adjacent concentric lamellae. Circumferential lamellae are arranged in parallel layers which enclose the entire bone. Osteocytic lacunae are seen.

three distinct layers: circumferential lamellae, concentric lamellae and interstitial lamellae. The *lamellae arranged in parallel layers* which enclose the entire bone at periosteal and endosteal surfaces are the *circumferential lamellae.* Deep to these circumferential lamellae, the *concentric lamellae* are arranged in the form of concentric layers *around a central vascular canal* known as *Haversian canal.* Each canal contains a capillary. This *Haversian canal with concentric lamellae* is known as *Haversian system or osteon* which is the basic metabolic unit of bone. There are approximately 4–20 concentric lamellae within each osteon and major bulk of compact bone is formed by concentric lamellae. *Haversian canals* of adjacent osteons are *joined by Volkmann canals* which contain blood vessels, thus having a rich vascular network to the compact bone. *Between* the *adjacent concentric lamellae, interstitial lamellae* are present and fill the spaces between them.

CANCELLOUS BONE (SPONGY BONE OR TRABECULAR BONE)

Cancellous bone consists of *long, slender trabeculae* (Fig. 7.4). These trabeculae show presence of osteocytes within them and osteoblasts or osteoclasts on the surface. These trabeculae *enclose wide marrow spaces* which are *filled by bone marrow. Bone marrow* is a *highly vascular tissue* which *provides nutrition to the bone.* In young bone, the marrow is red and haematopoietic. In old bone, there is loss of haemopoietic potential, the marrow is yellow and with increased accumulation of fat cells.

WOVEN BONE

Woven bone is the *first formed bone* with more irregular orientation of collagen fibres and with a variable diameter (Fig. 7.5). It is an *immature bone.* The collagen fibres are coarse and more in number. The *rate of formation* of bone is *more rapid* and has higher turnover rate. It shows

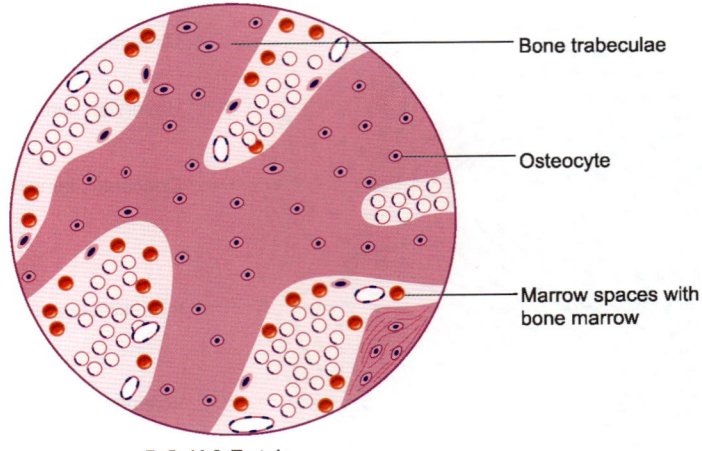

D.S. H & E stain

Figure 7.4   Cancellous bone – long slender bony trabeculae with osteocytes and wide marrow spaces.

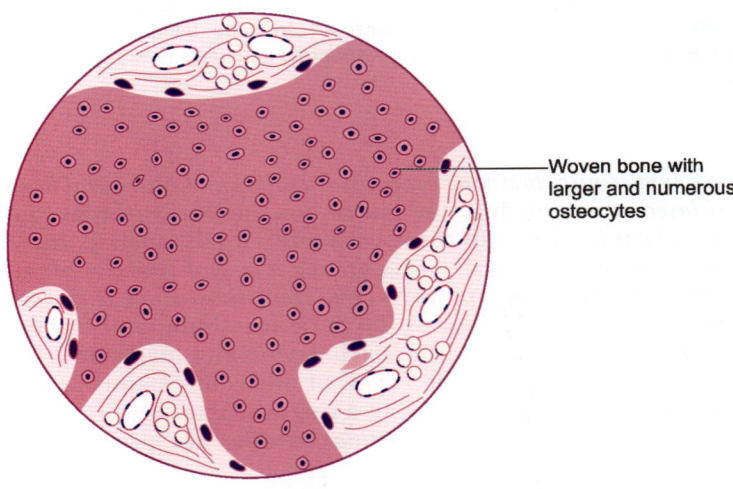

D.S. H & E stain

Figure 7.5   Woven bone – woven bone (immature bone) with larger and numerous osteocytes.

larger and more numerous cells, i.e. osteocytes and absence of lamellae or resting lines. It is seen during healing of fractures and healing of tooth sockets.

RESTING AND REVERSAL LINES

The lines that correspond to a *rest period* in continuous process of bone apposition are known as *resting lines* (Fig. 7.6). It has a more *regular appearance.*

Reversal lines (cement line) denote the *activity of bone from resorption* to deposition. These lines are *irregular* and appear strongly *basophilic* in H&E-stained sections due to high content of glycoprotein and proteoglycans (inorganic matrix) with little or no collagen. They appear irregular due to scalloped outline of Howship's lacunae.

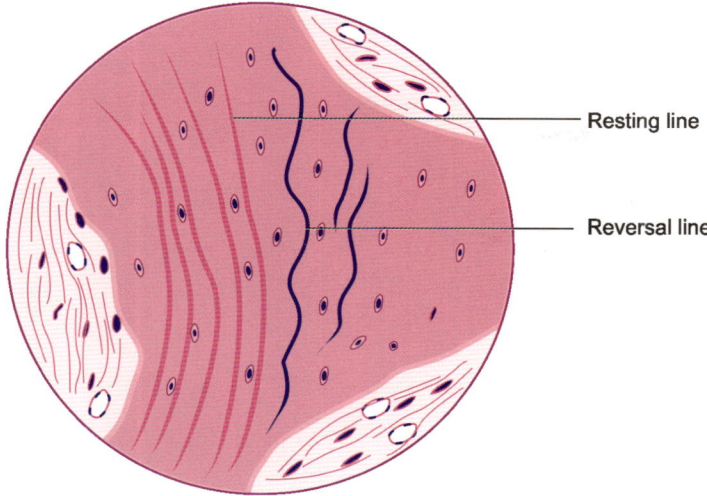

Figure 7.6 Resting and reversal lines – resting lines with regular appearance and reversal line with irregular and strongly basophilic appearance.

ALVEOLAR BONE PROPER

The *alveolar bone proper* is composed of *lamellated bone* and *bundle bone* (Fig. 7.7). It is *present around the root of the tooth* and gives attachment to the principal fibres of periodontal ligament.

Lamellated bone form *Haversian system* while some lamellae are roughly parallel to the surface of the adjacent marrow spaces. *Bundle bone* is that bone which *gives attachment to the principal fibres of periodontal ligament*. It contains few fibrils than the lamellated bone, so it *appears dark* in routine *H&E-stained sections*.

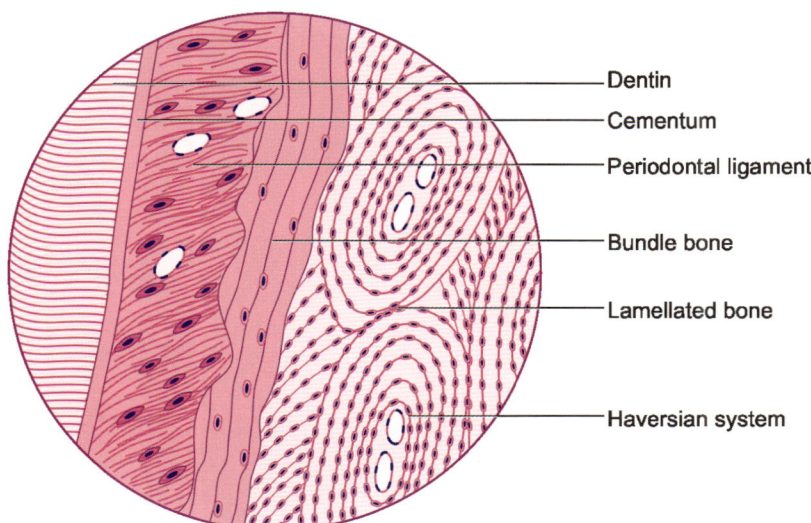

Figure 7.7 Alveolar bone proper – alveolar bone proper consisting of bundle bone and Haversian system.

Oral Mucous Membrane 8

GINGIVA

Gingiva is that part of the oral mucous membrane which surrounds the cervical region of tooth and the alveolar bone (which supports the roots of the teeth) (Fig. 8.1). It is the *region covered by masticatory mucosa*. Histologically, it shows thick *stratified squamous epithelium* which may be keratinized (15%) or nonkeratinized (10%), but *most often parakeratinized* (75%) (Fig. 8.2). The underlying *lamina propria* shows *dense connective tissue* with *long, slender and numerous connective tissue papillae* which consists of a dense network of closely packed collagen fibres. Some elastic fibres are also present. Few lymphocytes, plasma cells and macrophages are present in the connective tissue of normal gingiva adjacent to gingival sulcus. It is firmly attached to the underlying periosteum. It does not show large vessels but has long capillary loops. No distinct submucosa is seen.

GINGIVAL FIBRES

The lamina propria of gingiva consists of *dense collagen fibres* arranged in different groups:

i. Dentogingival fibres – these fibres extend from the *cervical cementum* into the *lamina propria of the gingiva*. These are the *most numerous* group of fibres.

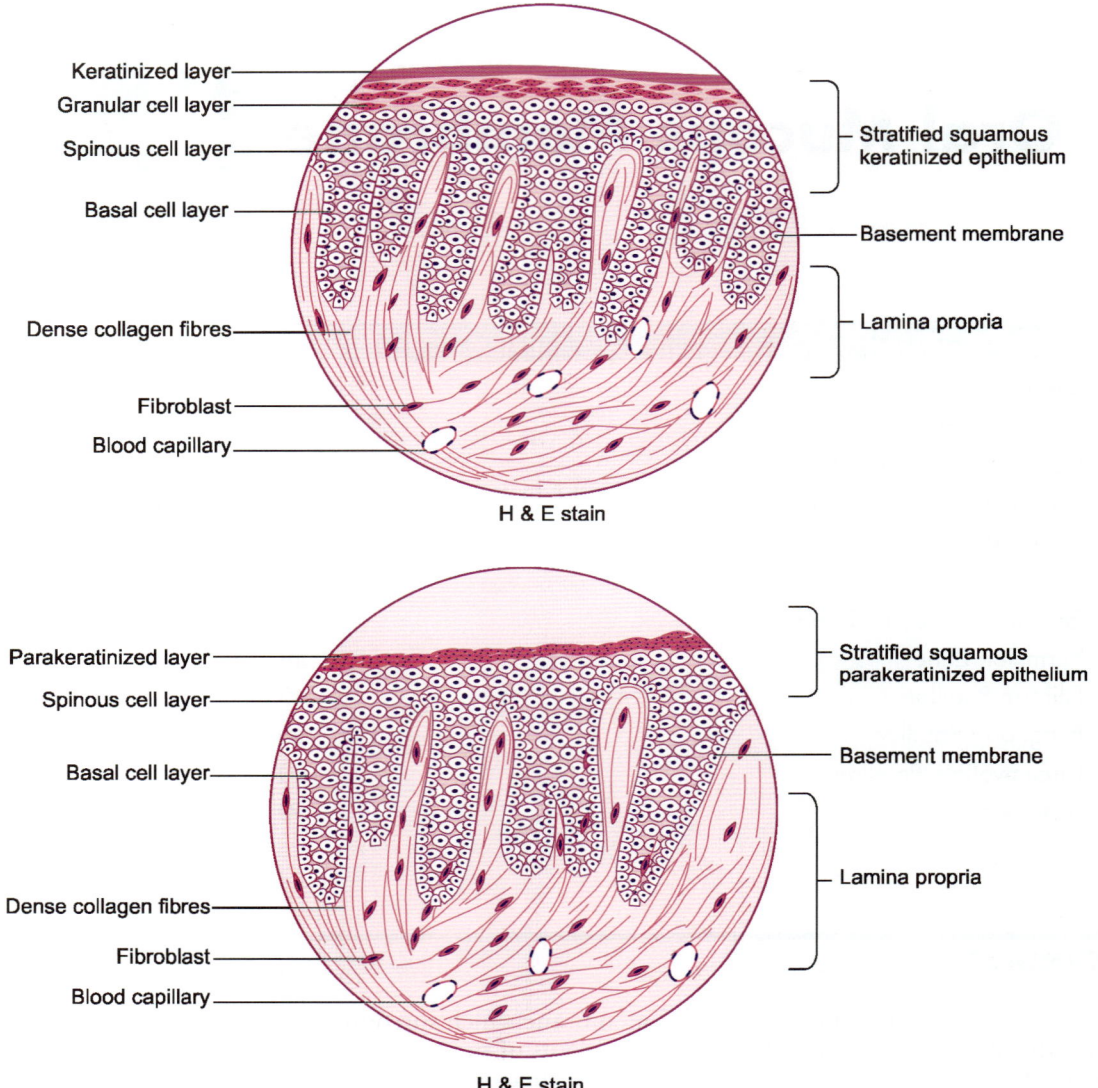

Figure 8.1 (A) Gingiva (keratinized) — gingiva covered by stratified squamous keratinized epithelium composed of basal cell layer resting on basement membrane, spinous cell layer, granular cell layer and superficial keratinized layer. The underlying lamina propria is dense with long, slender and numerous connective tissue papillae. (B) Gingiva (parakeratinized) — Gingiva covered by stratified squamous parakeratinized epithelium composed of basal cell layer resting on basement membrane, spinous cell layer, superficial keratin layer with pyknotic nuclei and indistinct granular cell layer. The underlying lamina propria is dense with long, slender and numerous connective tissue papillae.

ii. Alveologingival fibres – these fibres extend *from the alveolar crest* into the *lamina propria of the gingiva.*

iii. Circular fibres – these *fibres circle the tooth* and interlace with other group of fibres.

iv. Dentoperiosteal fibres – these fibres extend *from the cervical cementum to the periosteum of the alveolar crest, and of the vestibular and oral surfaces* of the *alveolar bone.*

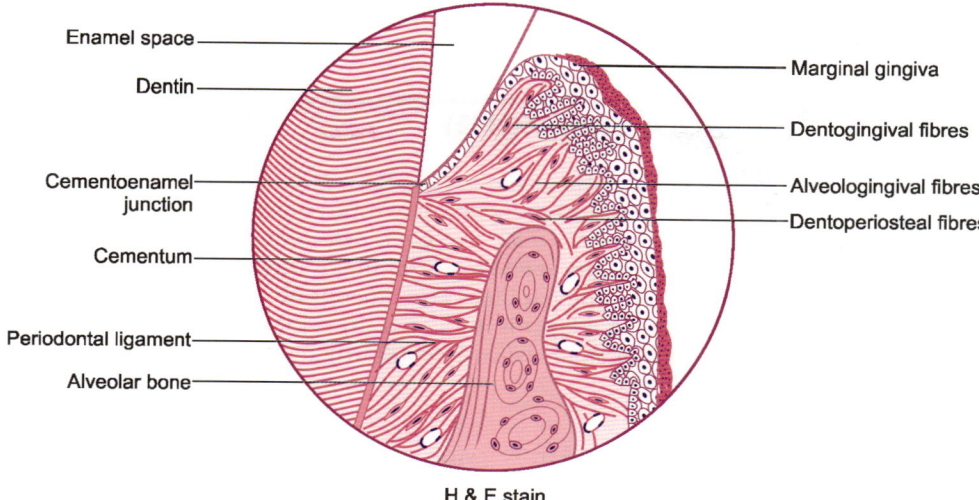

H & E stain

Figure 8.2   Gingival fibres – the lamina propria of the gingiva shows dentogingival, alveologingival and dentoperiosteal fibres of gingiva.

HARD PALATE (ANTEROLATERAL ZONE)

Hard palate is the region *covered by masticatory mucosa* (Fig. 8.3). *Anterolateral zone* or *fatty zone* is the area *between raphae and gingiva*. Histologically, it is *covered by thick, well keratinized stratified squamous epithelium*. The underlying *lamina propria* consists of a *dense connective tissue* that is thicker in the anterior part than the posterior part and has numerous long papillae. The mucous membrane is tightly fixed to the underlying periosteum. The submucosal layer is not generally evident. In the anterior zone, connective tissue shows the *presence of fat cells* which

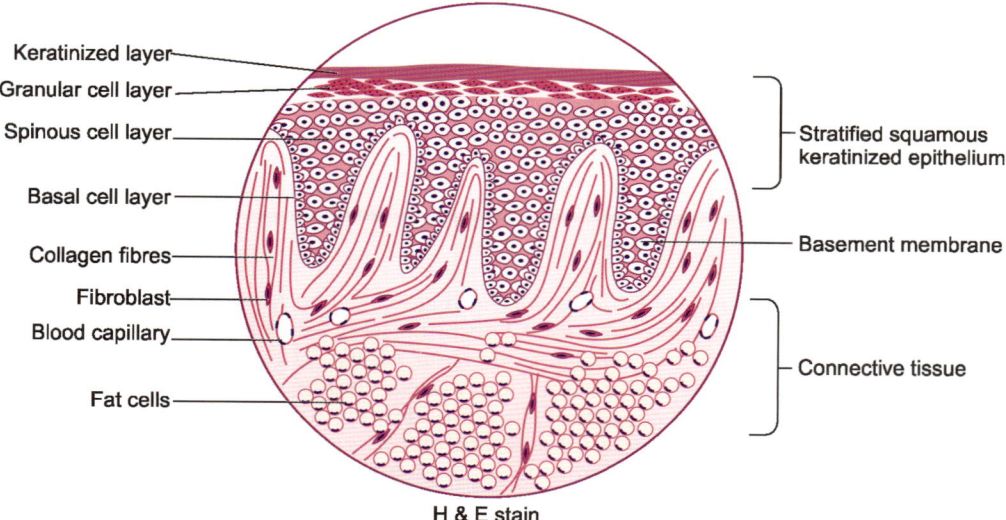

H & E stain

Figure 8.3   Hard palate (anterolateral zone) – hard palate covered by stratified squamous keratinized epithelium and underlying connective tissue with fat cells.

act as a cushion against the mechanical loads and protect the underlying nerves and blood vessels of the palate.

HARD PALATE (POSTEROLATERAL ZONE)

Hard palate is the region *covered by masticatory mucosa* (Fig. 8.4). *Posterolateral or glandular zone* is the *area between raphe and gingiva.* The fatty and the glandular zones meet in the region of first molar approximately. Histologically, it is *covered by thick, well keratinized stratified squamous epithelium.* The underlying *lamina propria* consists of a *dense connective tissue* that is thicker in the anterior part than the posterior part, and has numerous long papillae. The mucous membrane is tightly fixed to the underlying periosteum. The submucosal layer is not generally evident. In the posterior zone, the connective tissue shows the *presence of minor salivary glands* which are *mucous in nature* and act as cushion against the mechanical loads

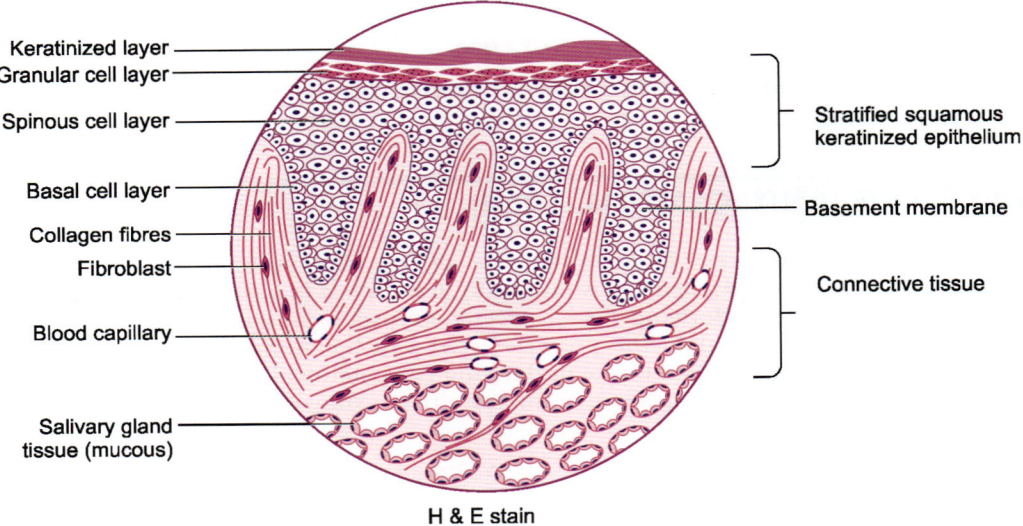

Keratinized layer
Granular cell layer
Spinous cell layer
Basal cell layer
Collagen fibres
Fibroblast
Blood capillary
Salivary gland tissue (mucous)

Stratified squamous keratinized epithelium
Basement membrane
Connective tissue

H & E stain

Figure 8.4   Hard palate (posterolateral zone) – hard palate covered by stratified squamous keratinized epithelium and underlying connective tissue with mucous salivary glands.

CHEEK MUCOSA

Cheek mucosa is the region *covered by lining mucosa* (Fig. 8.5). The *epithelium is thick nonkeratinized stratified squamous type* with *few wide rete ridges.* The underlying lamina propria consists of dense connective tissue with *short and irregular connective tissue papilla.* The connective tissue shows collagen fibres and also elastic fibres. The *submucosa is present* that firmly attaches the *lamina propria* to the underlying muscle tissue. It consists of strands of densely arranged collagen fibres. Between these strands, there is a loose connective tissue with *fat cells and many mixed minor salivary glands.* These glands are larger than those found in lip mucosa and usually present between bundles of buccinator muscles.

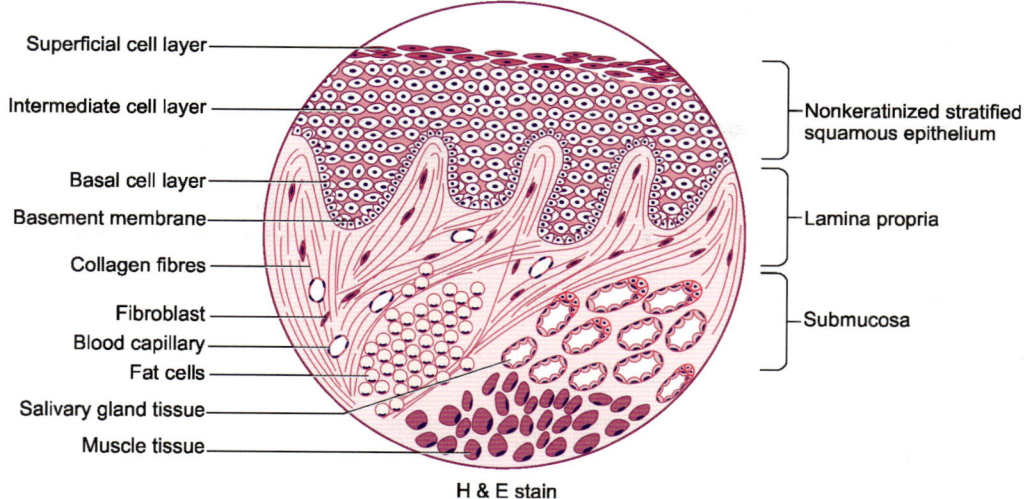

Superficial cell layer
Intermediate cell layer
Nonkeratinized stratified squamous epithelium
Basal cell layer
Basement membrane
Lamina propria
Collagen fibres
Fibroblast
Blood capillary
Submucosa
Fat cells
Salivary gland tissue
Muscle tissue

H & E stain

Figure 8.5 Cheek mucosa — cheek mucosa covered by non-keratinized stratified squamous epithelium composed of basal cell layer, intermediate cell layer and superficial cell layer. The lamina propria is seen with short papillae, submucosa with fat cells and mixed salivary gland tissue. Muscle tissue is also seen.

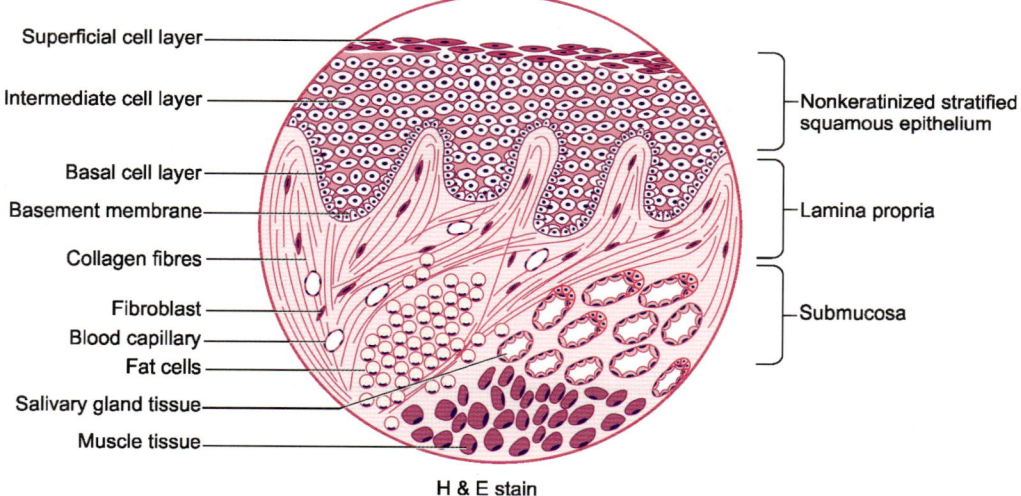

Superficial cell layer
Intermediate cell layer
Nonkeratinized stratified squamous epithelium
Basal cell layer
Basement membrane
Lamina propria
Collagen fibres
Fibroblast
Blood capillary
Submucosa
Fat cells
Salivary gland tissue
Muscle tissue

H & E stain

Figure 8.6 Lip mucosa — lip mucosa covered by non-keratinized stratified squamous epithelium composed of basal cell layer, intermediate cell layer and superficial cell layer. The lamina propria is seen with short papillae, submucosa with fat cells and mixed salivary gland tissue. Muscle tissue is also seen.

LIP MUCOSA

Lip mucosa is the *region covered by lining mucosa* (Fig. 8.6). The epithelium is *thick nonkeratinized stratified squamous type with few wide rete ridges.* The underlying lamina propria consists of dense connective tissue with *short and irregular connective tissue papillae.* The connective tissue shows collagen fibres and also elastic fibres. The *submucosa is present* that firmly attaches the lamina propria to the underlying orbicularis oris muscle. It consists of strands of densely arranged collagen fibres. Between these strands, there is a loose connective tissue with *fat cells and many mixed minor salivary glands.*

ECTOPIC SEBACEOUS GLAND

Isolated ectopic sebaceous glands are found in the *cheek mucosa lateral to the corner of the mouth and opposite to the molars* (Fig. 8.7). These are known as *Fordyce's spot*. Clinically they *appear as slightly elevated yellowish nodules*. They are not seen during childhood but the frequency increases with the advancing age. *Histologically* these *appear as typical sebaceous glands not associated with hair follicles.* The peripheral layer consists of flattened and darkly stained cells and the inner cells are pale, foamy with lipid rich cytoplasm. These glands have short keratinized ducts which open directly on the surface. Their role is not known. These are *not pathological lesions* but to be differentiated from pathological changes.

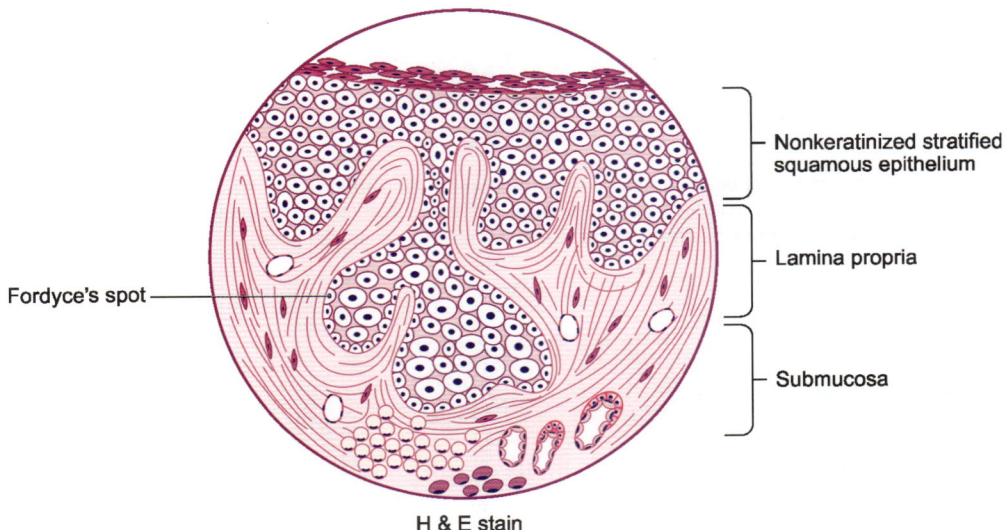

Nonkeratinized stratified squamous epithelium

Lamina propria

Submucosa

Fordyce's spot

H & E stain

Figure 8.7 Ectopic sebaceous glands (Fordyce's spots) – ectopic sebaceous glands found in the cheek mucosa. It consists of outermost small cells resting on basement membrane and innermost larger, more rounded cells filled with lipid.

VERMILION ZONE

Vermilion zone or red zone is the *transitional zone between the skin of the lip and the mucous membrane of the lip* (Fig. 8.8). It is *seen in the humans only*. The skin is separated from the vermilion zone by a line which is termed as vermilion border. The skin of the lip is covered by a moderately thick stratified squamous keratinized epithelium with a thick stratum corneum. The connective tissue papillae are few and short. Sebaceous glands in association with hair follicles and sweat glands are seen.

The *transitional region* is *covered by thin, orthokeratinized stratified squamous epithelium with numerous, densely arranged long papillae* of the lamina propria. These connective tissue papillae carry *large capillary loops* close to the surface of the epithelium. So, the blood is visible through thin parts of the translucent epithelium which *gives red colour to the lips*. This zone does not contain the salivary glands to keep it moist or to prevent it from drying as exposed to the atmosphere. Thus, the lips become dry easily and are licked to moisten.

The mucous membrane of the lip is covered by thick, nonkeratinized stratified squamous epithelium.

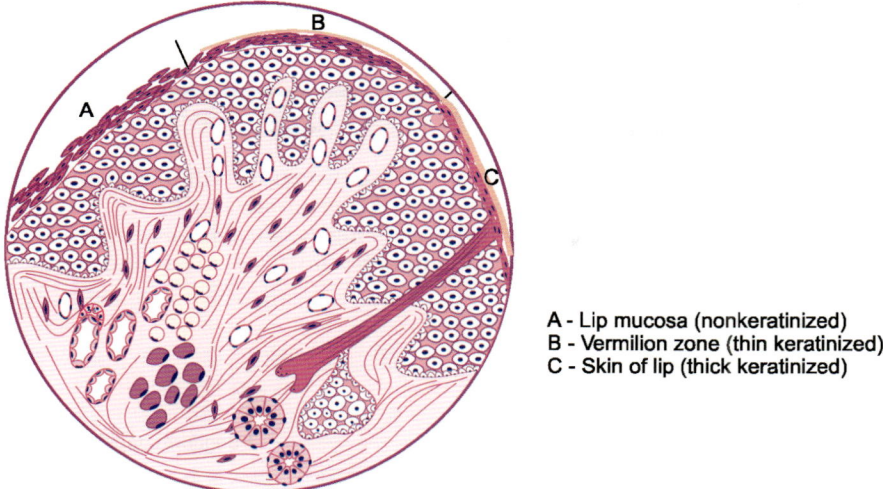

A - Lip mucosa (nonkeratinized)
B - Vermilion zone (thin keratinized)
C - Skin of lip (thick keratinized)

Figure 8.8   Vermilion zone — vermilion zone (A) is the transitional zone between the skin of the lip (C) and the mucous membrane of the lip (A). It is covered by orthokeratinized stratified squamous epithelium with long papillae having capillary loops close to the surface epithelium. Mucous membrane of the lip (A) is covered by non-keratinized stratified squamous epithelium. The skin of the lip (C) is covered by thick keratinized stratified squamous epithelium. Hair follicles, sebaceous glands and sweat glands are also seen.

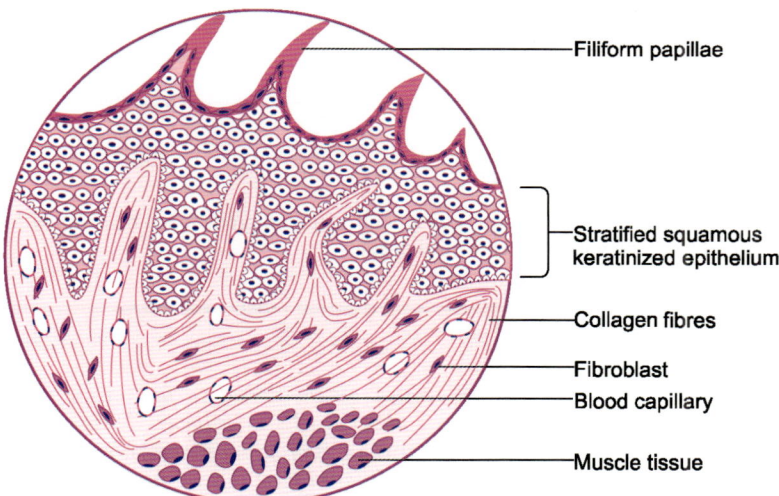

Filiform papillae

Stratified squamous
keratinized epithelium

Collagen fibres

Fibroblast
Blood capillary

Muscle tissue

Figure 8.9   Filiform papillae — filiform papillae as pointed conical projections covered by thick keratinized stratified squamous epithelium with a central core of connective tissue.

FILIFORM PAPILLAE

The *filiform papillae* appear as *numerous fine-pointed, cone-shaped structures* (hair like) covering most of the dorsal surface of anterior two-third part of the tongue (Fig. 8.9). These conical projections are epithelial structures *covered by a thick, keratinized stratified squamous epithelium* with a central core of connective tissue from which secondary papillae protrude toward the epithelium. These papillae *do not contain taste buds.*

FUNGIFORM PAPILLAE

Fungiform papillae are less numerous and interspersed between the filiform papillae and appear as *isolated, elevated mushroom-shaped smooth, round reddish prominences* on the *dorsal surface of anterior part of the tongue* (Fig. 8.10). They appear *red because of highly vascular connective tissue* covered by thin, nonkeratinized stratified squamous epithelium. *Few taste buds* are found in the epithelium *on the superior surface.*

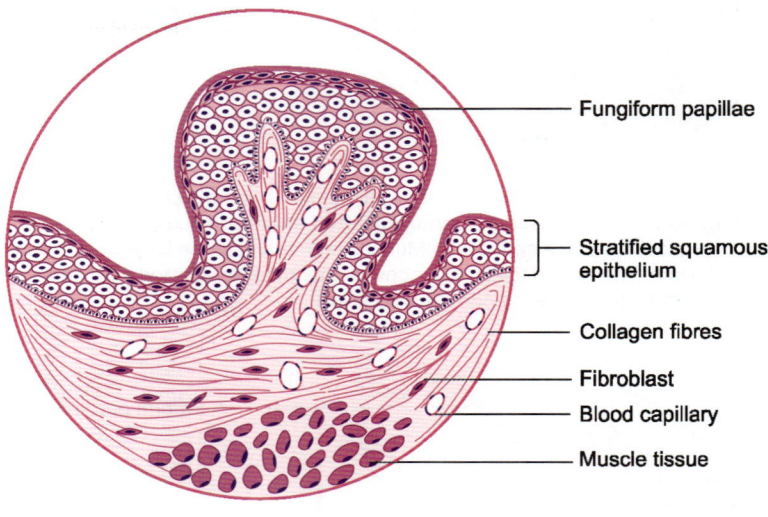

Fungiform papillae

Stratified squamous epithelium

Collagen fibres

Fibroblast

Blood capillary

Muscle tissue

H & E stain

Figure 8.10 Fungiform papillae – fungiform papilla as smooth rounded prominence covered by thin non-keratinized stratified squamous epithelium with vascular connective tissue.

CIRCUMVALLATE PAPILLAE

Circumvallate papillae (vallate papillae) are found *on the dorsal surface of the tongue adjacent and anterior to sulcus terminalis* (Fig. 8.11). They are about 8–12 in number. These are the largest papillae surrounded by a *deep circular groove* into which the *ducts of minor serous salivary glands* called as *von Ebner's glands open.* These are the *main source of salivary lipase.* These papillae are covered by keratinized stratified squamous epithelium with a connective tissue core. The epithelium shows presence of *numerous taste buds on the lateral surface.*

TASTE BUDS

Taste buds are *numerous around the walls of circumvallate papillae,* in the folds of foliate papillae, on the upper surface of fungiform papillae, in the mucosa of soft palate and in the epiglottis (Fig. 8.12). These are *small ovoid or barrel-shaped intraepithelial structures.* They *extend from the basal lamina* to *the surface of the epithelium.* Their *outer surface* is covered by a few flat epithelial cells which *surround a small opening* known as *taste pore.* These *taste buds* consist of *two types of cells — outer*

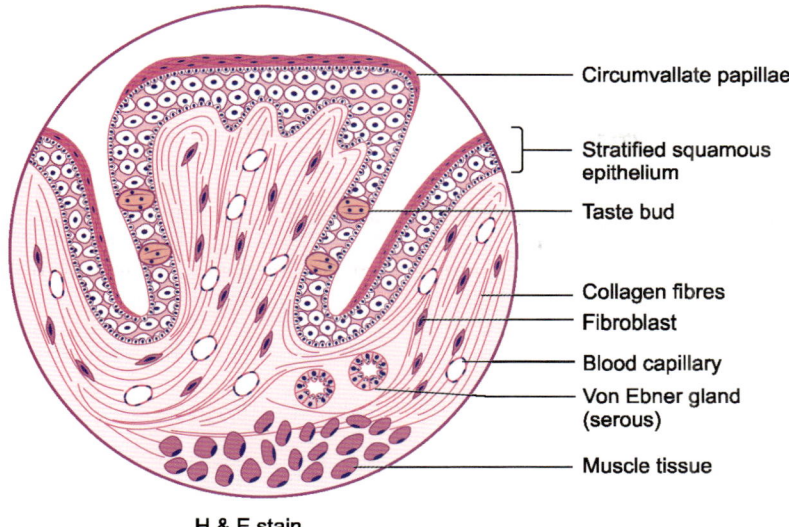

Circumvallate papillae

Stratified squamous epithelium

Taste bud

Collagen fibres

Fibroblast

Blood capillary

Von Ebner gland (serous)

Muscle tissue

H & E stain

Figure 8.11 Circumvallate papillae — circumvallate papilla is broader at the surface and covered by keratinized stratified squamous epithelium with taste buds on the lateral surface and von Ebner's gland which is serous in nature.

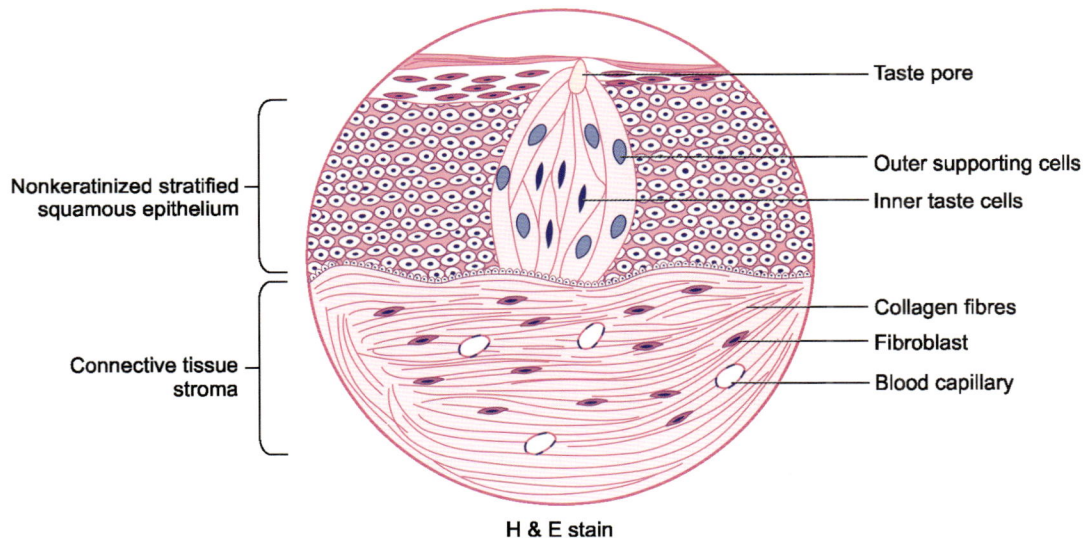

Taste pore

Outer supporting cells

Inner taste cells

Nonkeratinized stratified squamous epithelium

Collagen fibres

Fibroblast

Blood capillary

Connective tissue stroma

H & E stain

Figure 8.12 Taste buds – intraepithelial taste bud with taste pore, outer supporting cells and inner taste cells.

supporting cells and *inner taste cells*. The *outer supporting cells* are wider and *arranged like the staves of a barrel*. The *inner taste cells* are *shorter and spindle shaped*. Ten to 12 neuroepithelial cells are arranged between the taste cells which are the receptors of taste stimuli. These neuroepithelial cells are slender, dark staining cells with finger-like processes at their superficial end. These resemble like hairs at light microscopy. A rich nerve plexus is found below the taste buds.

Salivary Glands 9

Histologically, *salivary gland consists of* glandular secretory tissue, i.e. *parenchyma and the supporting connective tissue, i.e. stroma.* The parenchyma of major salivary gland is *surrounded by a capsule* which is composed of fibrous, vascular and neural tissues. *Fibrous septa* running inward from the capsule *divides the gland into major lobes,* and *lobes* are further *subdivided into lobules.* Each lobe contains *terminal secretory unit called acini.* This *secretory acinus* may be *serous, mucous or mixed* with central lumen. *Secretions from the acini get discharged into intercalated duct which are lined by a single layer of pale staining low cuboidal* cells. These are difficult to identity under light microscopy as they are compressed between secretory units. These *intercalated ducts join striated ducts* which are lined by a layer of tall columnar epithelial cells resting on a basement membrane. The cytoplasm of these cells is abundant and eosinophilic with large, centrally placed nucleus. The cytoplasm shows prominent striations. These *striated ducts join* each other *to form large excretory duct* lined by simple tall columnar epithelium or pseudostratified epithelium. Intercalated and striated ducts are intralobular (within the lobule) and excretory ducts are interlobular (within the connective tissue of lobules of gland).

The connective tissue components are mainly composed of collagen fibres with fibroblasts, macrophages, mast cells, occasional leucocytes, fat cells and plasma cells.

SEROUS ACINI

Serous cells are *pyramidal in shape* with a *broad base towards the basement membrane* and a *narrow apex towards the central lumen* (Fig. 9.1). These cells are smaller than mucous cells. The *nucleus* is spherical and *located* in the *basal third of the cell* or close to the base of the cell. In H&E-stained section, these cells have *basophilic cytoplasm* and *towards the apex of the cell,* there are numerous *deeply basophilic (dark purple) zymogen granules* which are secretory vesicles. These *granules* are *precursors of ptyalin.* Myoepithelial cells are seen at the periphery of the acini as stellate or spider-like cells but are difficult to identify in routine histology. Serous acini are generally spherical. Parotid gland is the pure serous gland.

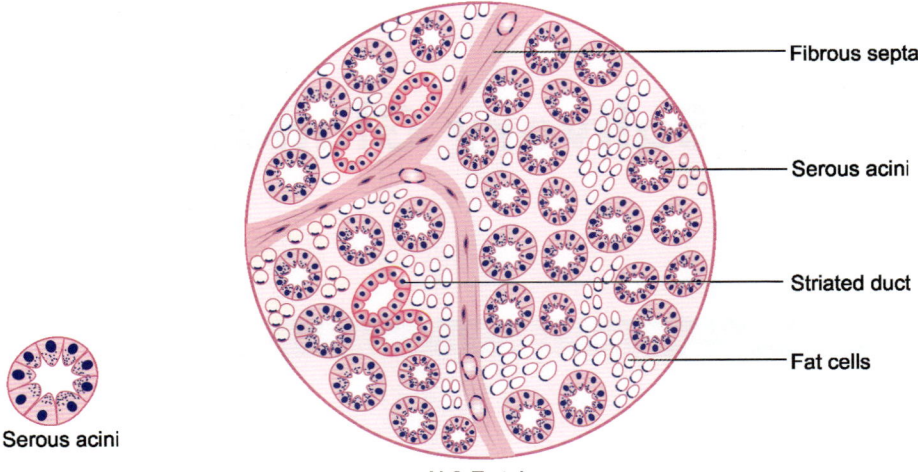

Serous acini

H & E stain

Figure 9.1   Serous acini – fibrous septa, secretory serous acini and striated ducts. Serous acini are generally spherical. Serous cells are pyramidal in shape with broad base and narrow apex. The spherical nucleus in basal region, basophilic cytoplasm and deeply basophilic zymogen granules. Striated ducts are lined by a layer of tall columnar epithelial cells with eosinophilic cytoplasm and centrally placed nucleus.

MUCOUS ACINI

Mucous cells are columnar *with a broad base resting on the basement membrane* (Fig. 9.2). The *cytoplasm* shows *presence of membrane-coated droplets of mucous* which gives it a *pale vacuolated appearance* as the mucinous content is not stained by routine stains or is lost during preparations. The *nucleus* is oval or flattened and *compressed against the base of the cell. Mucous acini* are generally *tubular.*

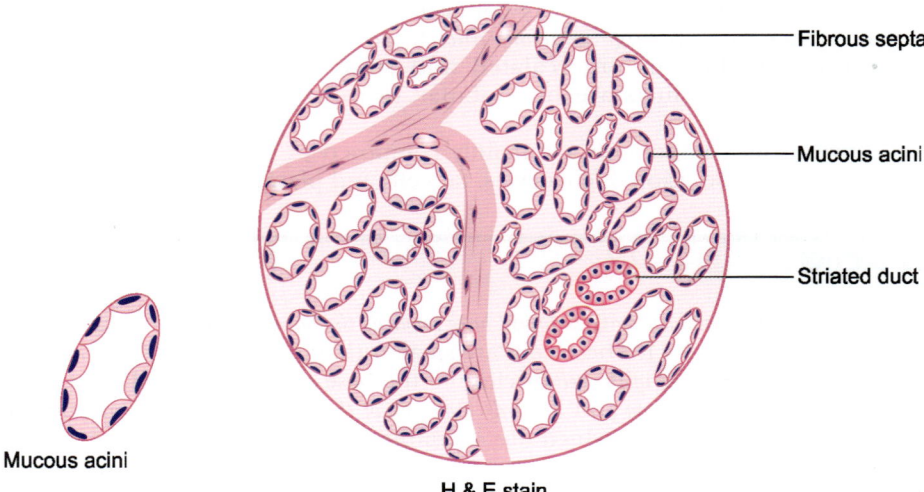

Mucous acini

H & E stain

Figure 9.2   Mucous acini — fibrous septa, secretory mucous acini and striated ducts. Mucous acini are generally tubular. Mucous cells are columnar with flattened nucleus compressed against the base of the cells and vacuolated appearance of cytoplasm. Striated ducts are lined by a layer of tall columnar epithelial cells with eosinophilic cytoplasm and centrally placed nucleus.

SEROUS CRESCENTS

In *mixed salivary glands*, the *proportion of serous and mucous cells vary* from *predominantly serous* as in human *submandibular gland* to *predominantly mucous* as in *human sublingual gland* (Fig. 9.3). Separate serous and mucous units may exist in addition to secretory units composed of both cell types. The *mucous cells* are *arranged in a tubular pattern* while the *serous cells* are present *at the blind ends of the tubules* in the *form of crescents or demilunes*. The secretion of the serous demilune cells reaches the lumen through intercellular canaliculi.

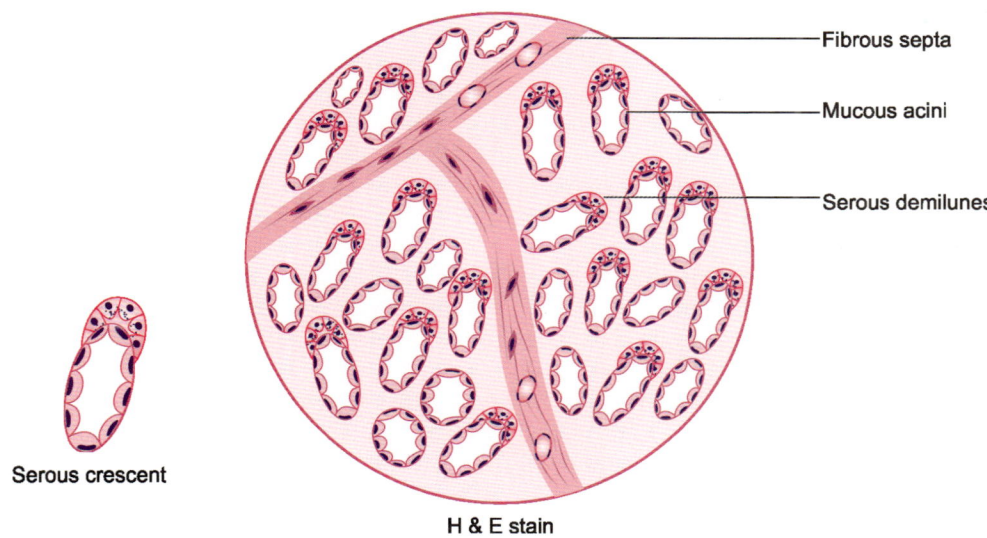

Serous crescent

Fibrous septa

Mucous acini

Serous demilunes

H & E stain

Figure 9.3 Serous crescents – fibrous septa and mucous acini with serous demilunes.

Maxillary Sinus

The maxillary sinus is one of the *largest paranasal sinuses* located *inside the body of maxilla* (Fig. 10.1). Histologically, it is lined by a mucosa which is firmly attached to the underlying periosteum. The *epithelium* is *pseudostratified ciliated columnar* type. In addition, it shows the presence of basal cells, columnar nonciliated cells and *mucus-secreting flask-shaped Goblet cells.* The underlying *connective tissue* is *composed of collagen fibres, fibroblasts, blood capillaries and nerve fibres.* In addition, *serous and mucous glands* are also *seen.*

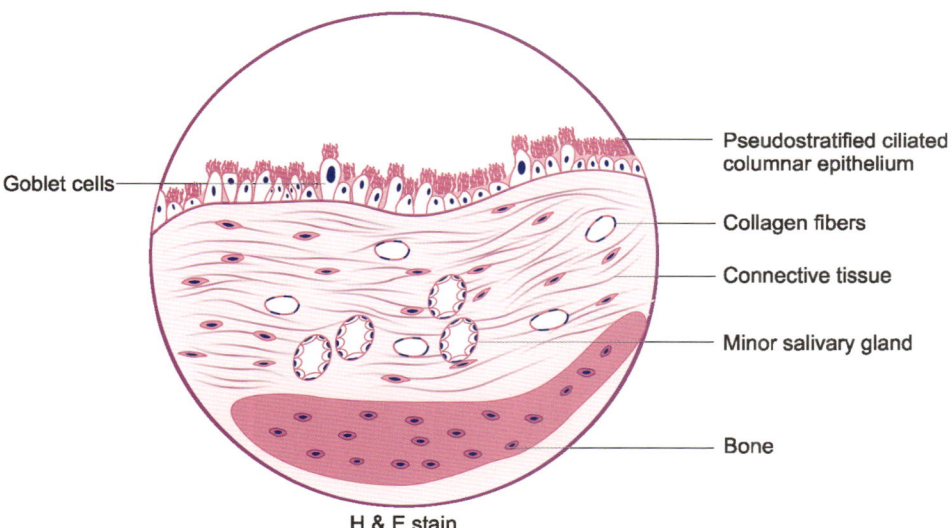

Goblet cells

Pseudostratified ciliated columnar epithelium

Collagen fibers

Connective tissue

Minor salivary gland

Bone

H & E stain

Figure 10.1 Maxillary sinus – maxillary sinus lined by pseudostratified ciliated columnar epithelium with goblet cells and the underlying connective tissue.

ORAL PATHOLOGY

SECTION 2

SECTION OUTLINE

Benign and Malignant Tumours of the Oral Cavity

11

BENIGN TUMOUR OF EPITHELIAL TISSUE ORIGIN

Squamous Papilloma

Squamous papilloma is a benign tumour of *epithelial tissue* characterized by *many, long finger-like projections* resulting in a *papillary* or *verruciform mass* (Fig. 11.1). It consists of *proliferation* of *stratified squamous epithelium* with a *thin central core of connective tissue*. There may be

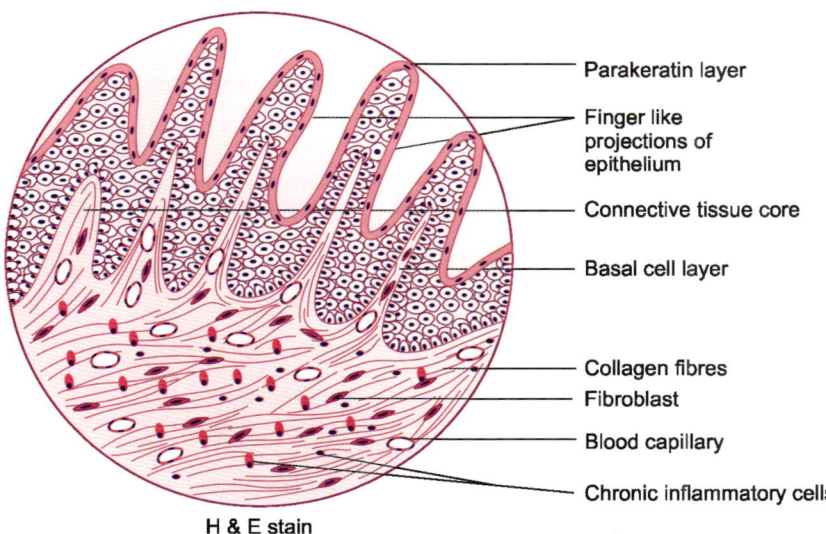

Parakeratin layer

Finger like projections of epithelium

Connective tissue core

Basal cell layer

Collagen fibres

Fibroblast

Blood capillary

Chronic inflammatory cells

H & E stain

Figure 11.1 Squamous papilloma — many long, finger-like projections with a thin core of connective tissue.

hyperkeratosis. *Proliferation of spinous cell layer* (acanthosis) is an *essential feature*. The fibrovascular connective tissue stroma may show the presence of chronic inflammatory cells. Koilocytes, HPV (human papilloma virus) altered epithelial clear cells (with small dark nuclei and perinuclear clear space) are sometimes seen in upper part of the spinous cell layer.

POTENTIALLY MALIGNANT DISORDERS

Leukoplakia

Leukoplakia is the *most common potentially malignant lesion* of the oral mucosa and is a descriptive clinical term by exclusion of other white lesions (Fig. 11.2A). Histologically, it shows *hyperkeratosis* of surface *layer* and *epithelial hyperplasia*. The surface layer may show hyperparakeratosis or hyperorthokeratosis or a combination of both. In hyperparakeratosis, there is no granular cell

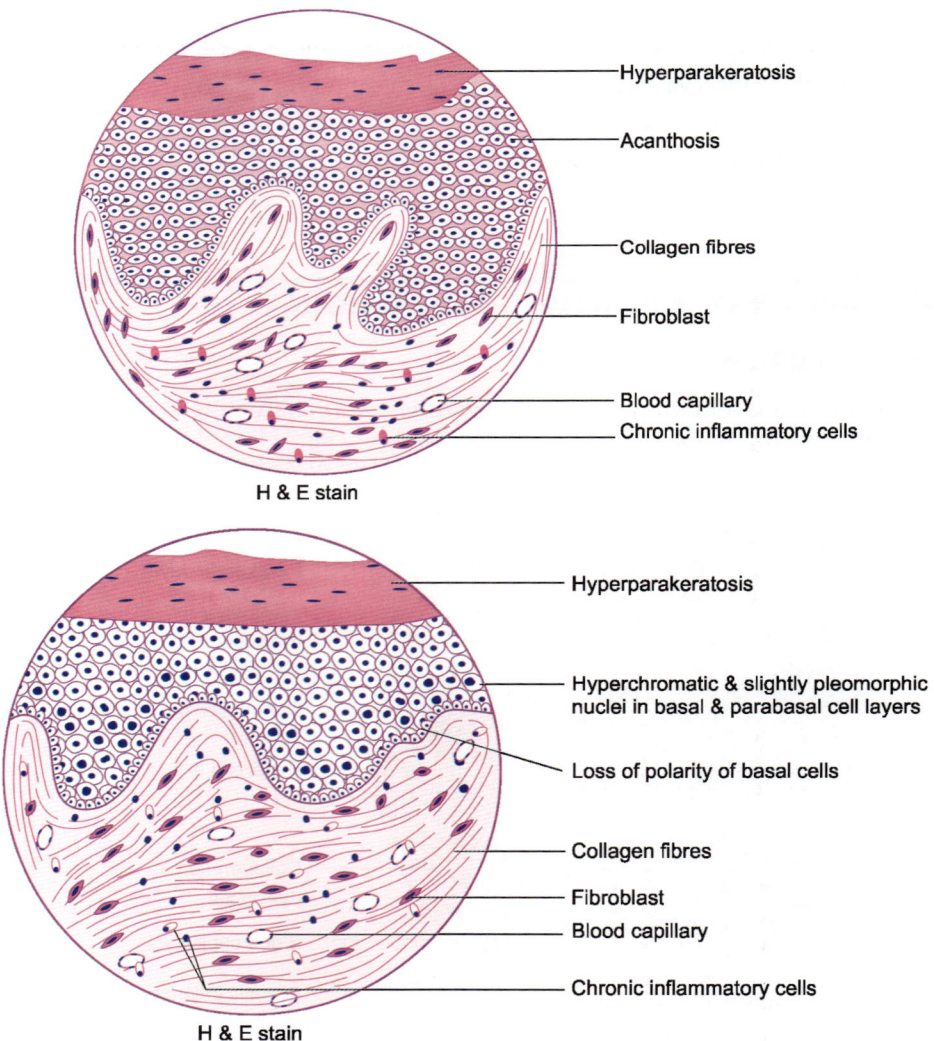

Figure 11.2   (A) Hyperkeratosis (leukoplakia) — hyperkeratosis of surface layer with epithelial hyperplasia. (B) Mild epithelial dysplasia — dysplastic features are seen in basal and parabasal cell layers of the epithelium.

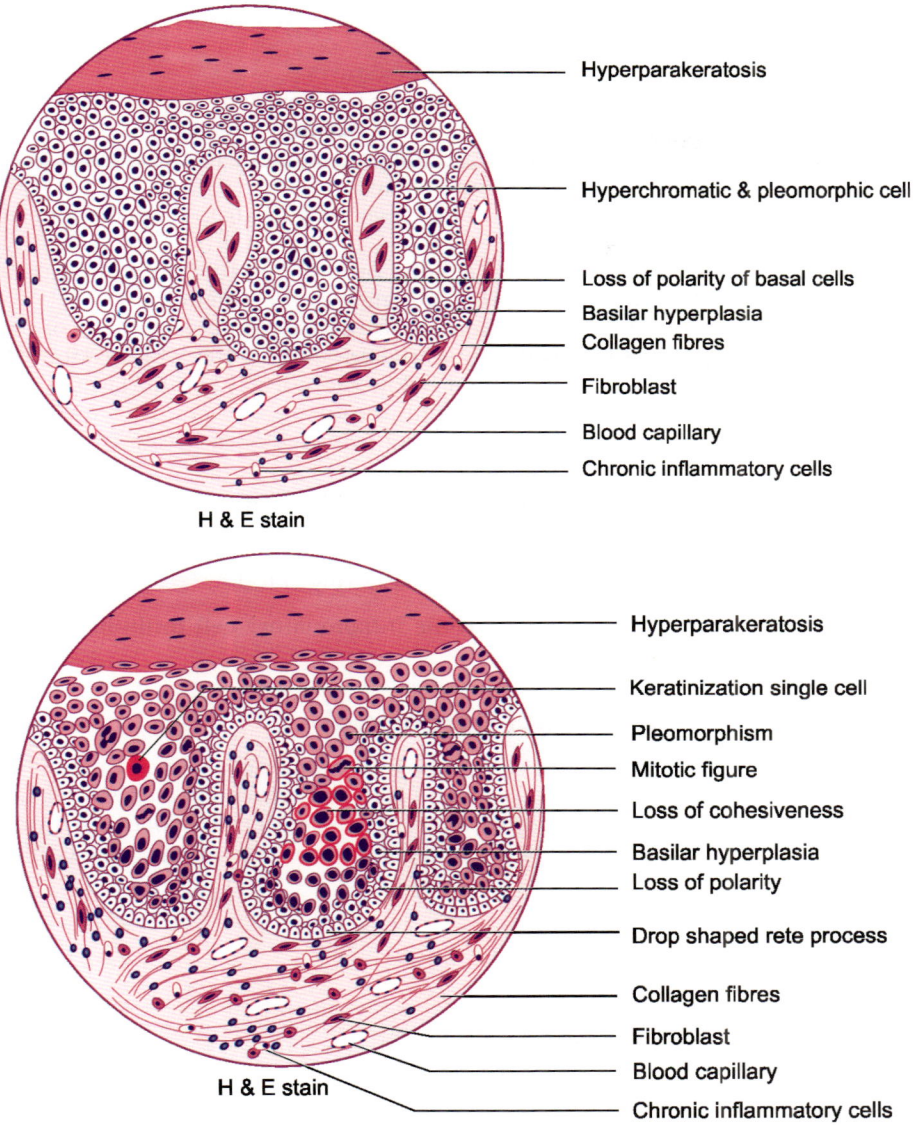

Figure 11.2, cont'd   (C) Moderate epithelial dysplasia — dysplastic features are seen from basal cell layer to the midportion of spinous cell layer. (D) Severe epithelial dysplasia — dysplastic features are seen from basal cell layer to a level above the midpoint of the epithelium.

layer and nuclei are seen in the keratin layer. In hyperorthokeratinization, there is a prominent granular cell layer and nuclei are lost in the keratin layer.

Epithelial dysplasia (abnormality of development), if present, is graded subjectively as *mild, moderate and severe.*

Following are the features of epithelial dysplasia:

  i. Enlarged cells and nuclei.
 ii. Cellular and nuclear pleomorphism: Variation in size and shape of cells and nuclei.
iii. Hyperchromatism of nuclei: Excessive dark staining of nuclei due to increased DNA synthesis.

iv. Increased nuclear to cytoplasmic ratio: Size of the nucleus is increased in relation to the cytoplasm.
v. Large and prominent nucleoli.
vi. Increased mitosis: Increase in number of mitotic figures.
vii. Abnormal mitosis: Mitotic figures in various forms other than normal in any layer of the epithelium superficial to basal cell layer, e.g. tripolar mitotic figure.
viii. Loss of cohesiveness of cells: The cells lose their attachment to the adjacent cells due to faulty or reduced attachment of their desmososmes.
ix. Bulbous or teardrop-shaped rete ridges: Rete pegs become drop-shaped wider at the base than superficial.
x. Loss of polarity: The basal cells lose their cellular orientation; they are not perpendicular to the epithelial connective junction but are at an angle to the junction.
xi. Irregular stratification of epithelium: There is disturbance in arrangement of cells as they pass from basal cell layer to the surface, thus affecting the regular stratification pattern.
xii. Abnormal keratinization: Keratin is formed below the normal keratin layer. There may be keratin pearl formation or individual cell keratinization.
- If the dysplastic features are seen in *basal and parabasal layer*, it is *mild epithelial dysplasia* (Fig. 11.2B).
- If the *dysplastic features* are seen from *basal cell layer* to midportion of spinous cell layer, it is *moderate epithelial dysplasia* (Fig. 11.2C).
- If the dysplastic features are seen from the basal cell layer to a level above the midpoint of the epithelium, it is severe epithelial dysplasia (Fig. 11.2D).

The underlying connective tissue shows chronic inflammatory cell infiltration (lymphocytes and plasma cells) of variable intensity.

Carcinoma In Situ (Intraepithelial Carcinoma)

Carcinoma in situ is a condition which occurs on mucous membrane of oral cavity (Fig. 11.3). It has a variable histologic appearance but *characterized by top to bottom epithelial dysplasia*, i.e. *dysplastic features* extending from *basal layer to the surface of the epithelium*. All the dysplastic features are confined to the epithelium without invasion of the underlying connective tissue. The epithelium may

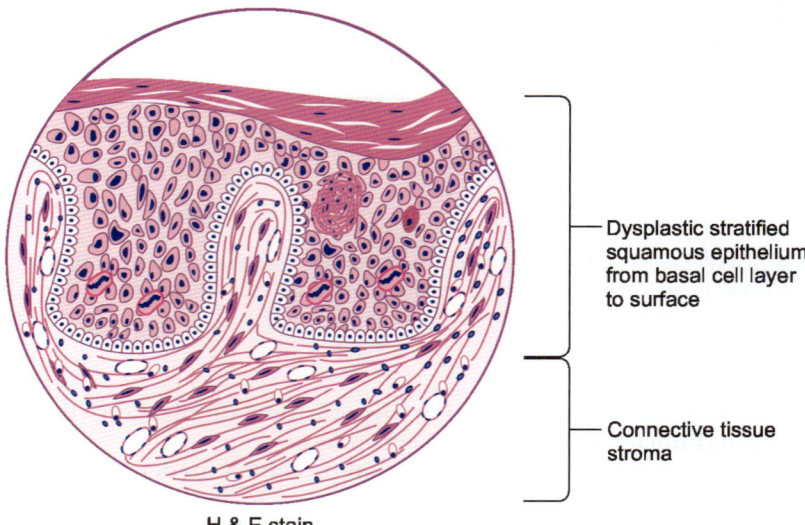

Dysplastic stratified squamous epithelium from basal cell layer to surface

Connective tissue stroma

H & E stain

Figure 11.3 Carcinoma in situ — dysplastic features extending from basal cell layer to the surface of the epithelium without invasion of underlying connective tissue.

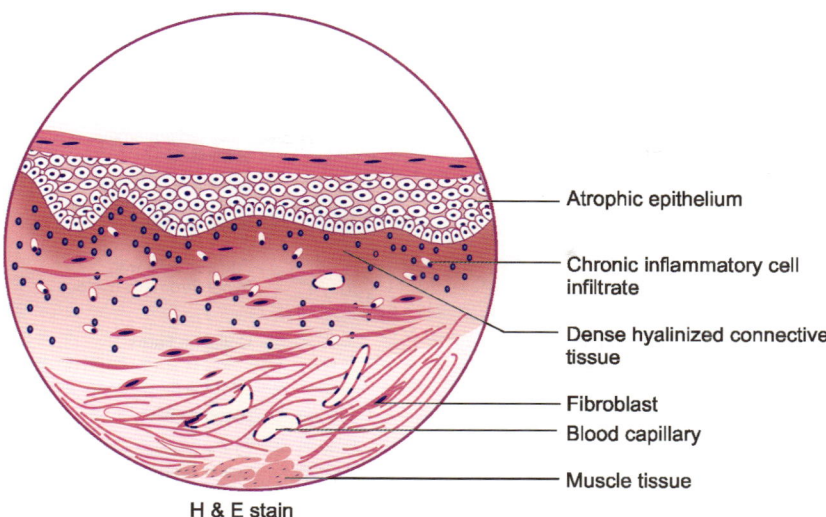

H & E stain

Figure 11.4   Oral submucous fibrosis — atrophic epithelium and dense hyalinized connective tissue stroma with chronic inflammatory cell infiltration.

be atrophic or hyperplastic. Chronic inflammatory cell infiltration in the connective tissue is a variable finding.

Oral Submucous Fibrosis

Oral submucous fibrosis is a *chronic, progressive, potentially malignant disorder* of the oral mucosa (Fig. 11.4). The *overlying epithelium* shows *hyperkeratosis* and/or *atrophy* depending on the different stages of the lesion. Epithelial dysplasia may be seen. The underlying connective tissue shows dense hyalinized *hypovascular collagenous stroma* with *variable number of chronic inflammatory cells,* mainly lymphocytes and plasma cells.

MALIGNANT TUMOURS OF EPITHELIAL TISSUE ORIGIN

Basal Cell Carcinoma (Basal Cell Epithelioma, Rodent Ulcer)

Basal cell carcinoma is a skin cancer and is believed to *arise from the basal cell layer of skin* (pluripotential stem cell compartments of basal cell layer of epidermis) and its appendages (Fig. 11.5). It does not arise in the oral mucosa and, thus *occurs in the oral cavity by invasion and infiltration from a skin surface.* Histologically, it has a varied appearance depending on the clinical subtypes. Typically it shows *tumour cells arranged in well-demarcated islands, nests or strands of varying size.* The tumour cells are *uniform, ovoid basaloid cells* with *hyperchromatic nuclei* and with *relatively less cytoplasm.* The *epithelial islands show palisading of the peripheral cells.* Some connection with the overlying epidermis may be seen in early lesions. Clear zone of retraction artefact is seen between the epithelial islands and the connective tissue. Increased mucin is frequently seen in the surrounding stroma.

Squamous Cell Carcinoma (Epidermoid Carcinoma)

Squamous cell carcinoma is the most *common malignant neoplasm of oral cavity* of *epithelial tissue origin* (Fig. 11.6). It arises from overlying dysplastic surface epithelium. Histologically, it shows *epithelial*

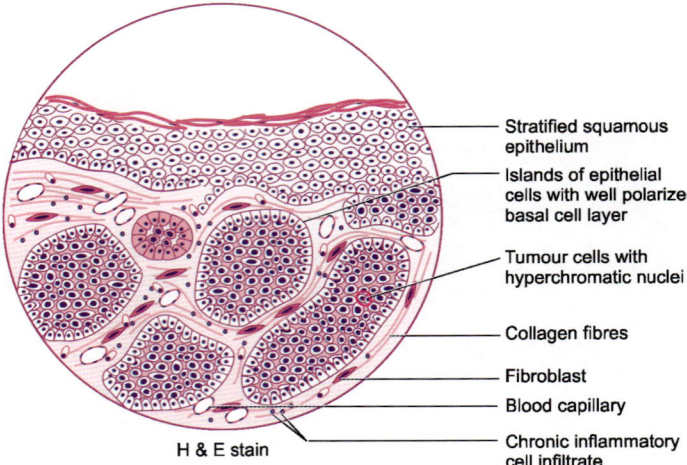

Stratified squamous epithelium

Islands of epithelial cells with well polarized basal cell layer

Tumour cells with hyperchromatic nuclei

Collagen fibres

Fibroblast

Blood capillary

Chronic inflammatory cell infiltrate

H & E stain

Figure 11.5   Basal cell carcinoma – invaded islands of epithelial cells with well-polarized peripheral basal cell layer and uniform, ovoid tumour cells with hyperchromatic nuclei.

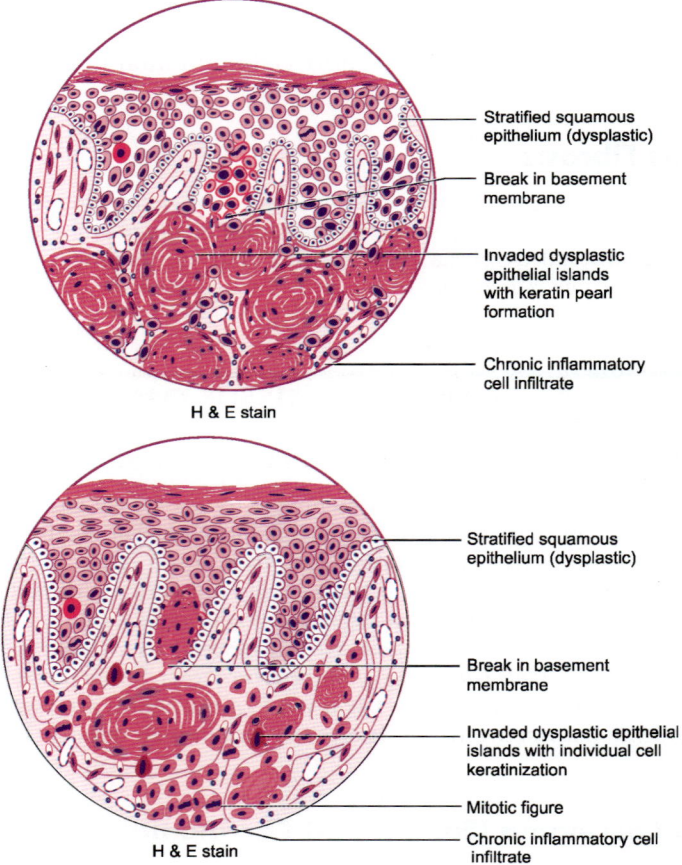

Stratified squamous epithelium (dysplastic)

Break in basement membrane

Invaded dysplastic epithelial islands with keratin pearl formation

Chronic inflammatory cell infiltrate

H & E stain

Stratified squamous epithelium (dysplastic)

Break in basement membrane

Invaded dysplastic epithelial islands with individual cell keratinization

Mitotic figure

Chronic inflammatory cell infiltrate

H & E stain

Figure 11.6   (A) Squamous cell carcinoma – well differentiated – break in the continuity of the basement membrane with invasion of dysplastic epithelial islands in the underlying lamina propria with keratin pearl formation. (B) Squamous cell carcinoma – moderately differentiated – invasion of dysplastic epithelial cells with individual cell keratinization and marked variation in size, shape and staining characteristics.

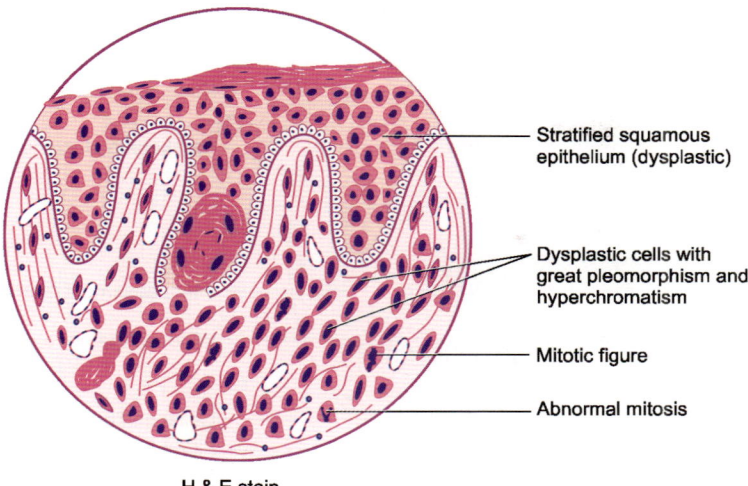

Stratified squamous
epithelium (dysplastic)

Dysplastic cells with
great pleomorphism and
hyperchromatism

Mitotic figure

Abnormal mitosis

H & E stain

Figure 11.6, cont'd   (C) Squamous cell carcinoma – poorly differentiated – marked pleomorphism and hyperchromatism of dysplastic cells with no keratin formation and numerous mitotic figures.

proliferation and *invasion of underlying connective tissue by sheets, islands or cords of dysplastic epithelial cells.* Lesion is graded as well-differentiated squamous cell carcinoma, moderately differentiated squamous cell carcinoma and poorly differentiated squamous cell carcinoma according to the degree to which the tumour resembles the parent tissue, i.e. squamous epithelium, and production of its normal product, i.e. keratin.

Well-Differentiated Squamous Cell Carcinoma

It consists of sheets and nests of *dysplastic epithelial cells* (Fig. 11.6A). These *cells are large with abundant eosinophilic cytoplasm, hyperchromatic* (darkly staining) *nuclei* and *increased nuclear cytoplasmic ratio.* Cellular and nuclear pleomorphism is of variable degrees. *Formation of numerous epithelial* or keratin *pearls of varying size* (a round focus of concentrically layered keratinized cells) is one of the most *prominent feature.* Single cell may also undergo individual cell keratinization. Mitotic figures may be seen. The *adjacent connective tissue shows marked chronic inflammatory cell response.*

Moderately Differentiated Squamous Cell Carcinoma

It shows a *greater variability* in histologic pattern (Fig. 11.6B). There is a *marked variation in cell size, shape and staining characteristics. Mitotic activity* is often *very prominent* with both normal and abnormal forms. Keratin pearl may be present but not a prominent feature. *Individual cell keratinization* is commonly noticed. There is moderate *chronic inflammatory cell response.*

Poorly Differentiated Squamous Cell Carcinoma

It bears less *resemblance* to the *cell of origin* (Fig. 11.6C). There is *little or no keratin formation.* The *neoplastic cells* show *extreme degrees of pleomorphism* and *hyperchromatism* with *many normal and abnormal mitotic figures.* Tumour giant cells may be seen. There is *minimal chronic inflammatory cell response.*

Verrucous Carcinoma

Verrucous carcinoma is a low *grade variant of oral squamous cell carcinoma* (Fig. 11.7). It is *characterized by exophytic overgrowth* of *well-differentiated stratified squamous epithelium with papillary surface.* It shows

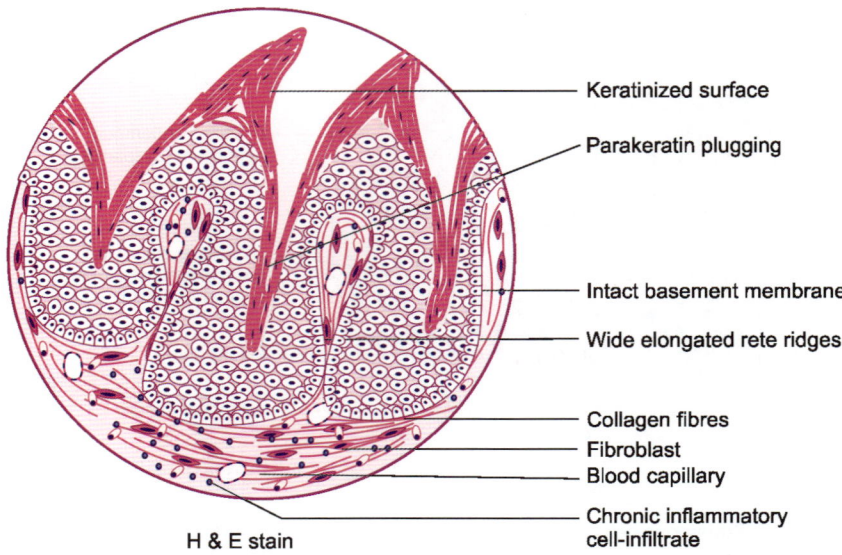

Keratinized surface

Parakeratin plugging

Intact basement membrane

Wide elongated rete ridges

Collagen fibres

Fibroblast

Blood capillary

Chronic inflammatory cell-infiltrate

H & E stain

Figure 11.7   Verrucous carcinoma — exophytic overgrowth of well-differentiated stratified squamous epithelium with papillary surface. Wide rete ridges with parakeratin plugging and intact basement membrane is evident.

wide, elongated rete ridges with *pushing borders* into the underlying connective tissue. *Cleft-like spaces* with a *thick layer of parakeratin extend from the surface* deeply into the lesion (*parakeratin plugging*). There is *no cellular atypia* or sometimes if present it may be minimal. The *basement membrane often appears to be intact.* There is intense chronic inflammatory cell infiltration in the adjacent connective tissue.

Malignant Melanoma

It is an *uncommon neoplasm of melanocytes* (Fig. 11.8). These cells may be *round* or *spindle* shaped or both.

The *intraepithelial component*, i.e. *radial growth phase* is characterized by the *presence of large, epithelioid melanocytes* along the *epithelial mesenchymal junction. Vertical growth phase* is characterized by *invasion* and *proliferation of malignant epithelioid melanocytes* in the *underlying connective tissues.* These cells may be arranged singly or in clusters and *often show presence of melanin granules.* There is chronic inflammatory cell response.

BENIGN TUMOURS OF CONNECTIVE TISSUE ORIGIN

Fibroma

Fibroma is the *most common benign connective* tissue *tumour of the oral cavity* (Fig. 11.9). Mostly it is a *reactive hyperplasia of fibrous connective tissue* in response to local irritation or trauma. Histologically, it *shows* radiating, *circular or irregularly arranged interlacing bundles of collagen fibres* with *variable number of fibroblasts or fibrocytes.* The *overlying stratified squamous* epithelium is *atrophic* due to the underlying fibrous tissue. There may be hyperkeratosis of the surface epithelium due to secondary trauma. Chronic inflammatory cell infiltration of lymphocytes and plasma cells may be seen.

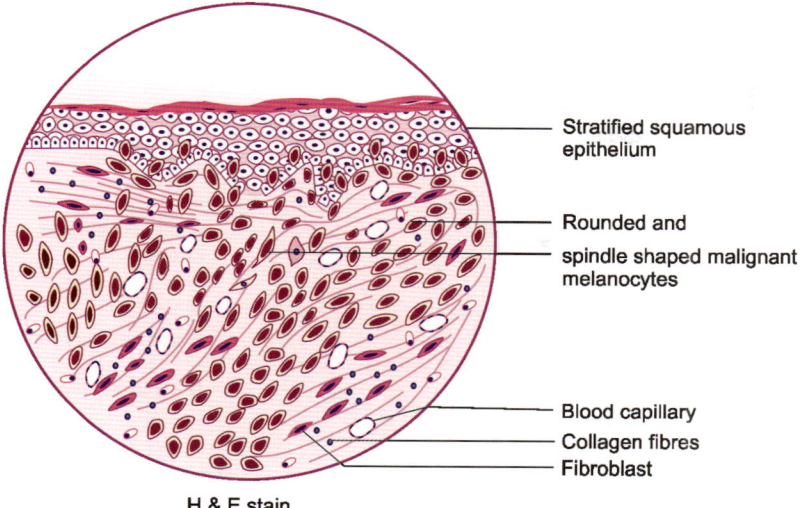

Stratified squamous epithelium

Rounded and spindle shaped malignant melanocytes

Blood capillary
Collagen fibres
Fibroblast

H & E stain

Figure 11.8 Malignant melanoma – malignant melanocytes which may be rounded or spindle shaped.

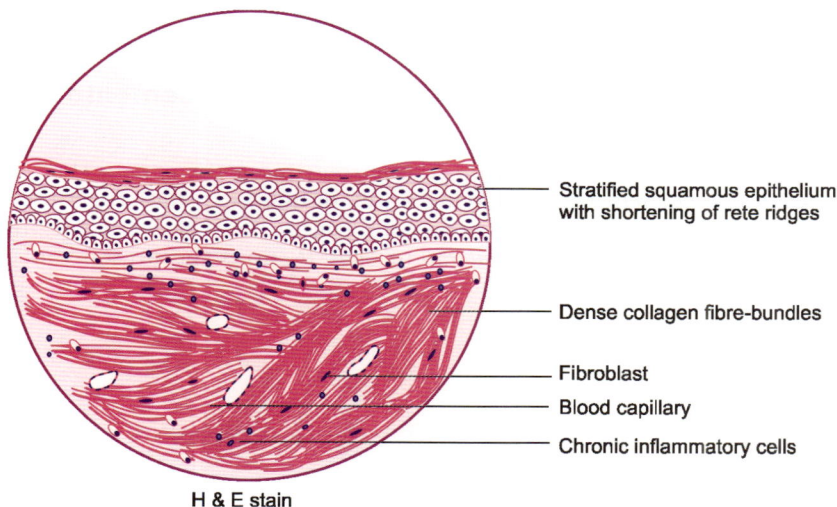

Stratified squamous epithelium with shortening of rete ridges

Dense collagen fibre-bundles

Fibroblast
Blood capillary
Chronic inflammatory cells

H & E stain

Figure 11.9 Fibroma – interlacing bundles of collagen fibres and overlying stratified squamous epithelium with shortening of rete ridges.

Peripheral Ossifying Fibroma (Peripheral Cementifying Fibroma, Peripheral Fibroma with Calcification, Ossifying Fibroid Epulis)

Peripheral ossifying fibroma is considered to be a *reactive lesion* rather than a neoplastic lesion, *occurring mostly on the gingiva* (Fig. 11.10). The *lesional tissue* is covered *by intact stratified squamous epithelium.* Sometimes it may be ulcerated. The *underlying connective tissue* is composed of *fibrous proliferation* and a *cellular connective tissue* with *large number of proliferating fibroblasts.* The *calcified component* is of variable amounts and may be *bone, or osteoid, cementum-like material* or *dystrophic calcifications.* Dystrophic calcifications are in the form of small globules, granules or large, irregular areas of basophilic calcified material.

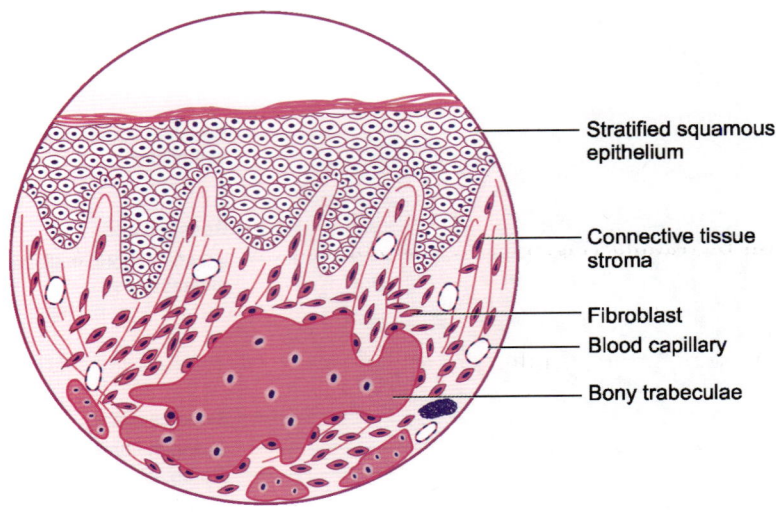

H & E stain

Figure 11.10   Peripheral ossifying fibroma — intact stratified squamous epithelium and cellular fibrous connective tissue stroma with irregular trabeculae of bone.

Central Ossifying Fibroma (Cementifying Fibroma, Cemento-ossifying Fibroma)

Central ossifying fibroma is a *benign central (intraosseous) neoplasm of bone* (Fig. 11.11). Histologically, the *lesion is well circumscribed* (having a well-defined capsule) from the surrounding bone. The appearance is variable. It is *composed of fibrous tissue* with *variable degrees of cellularity containing bony trabeculae, cementum-like material* or *both*. It shows the presence of many *delicate*

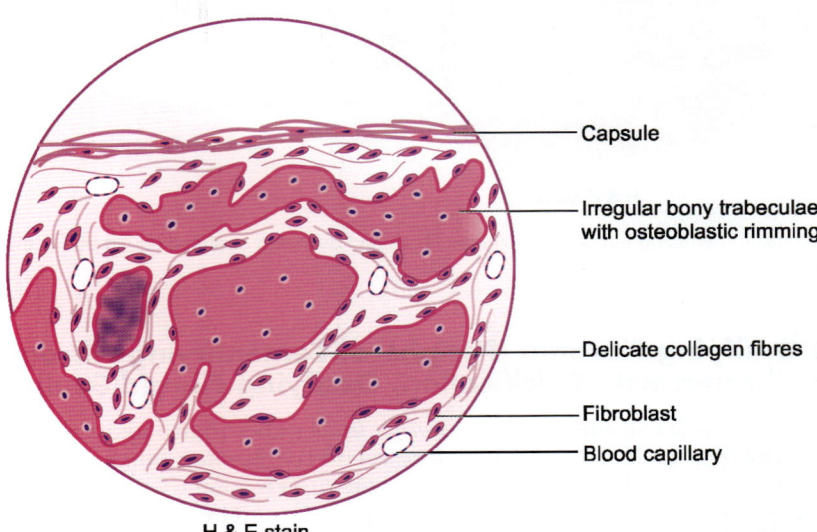

H & E stain

Figure 11.11   Central ossifying fibroma — well-circumscribed lesion with irregular bony trabeculae having osteoblastic rimming and delicate collagen fibres.

interlacing collage fibres interspersed with proliferating fibroblasts. The mineralized component may be in form of osteoid, bone, cementum-like material or in a combination ranging from scanty to large amount. The bony *trabeculae vary* in size and show *peripheral osteoid and osteoblastic rimming.*

Peripheral Giant Cell Granuloma (Giant Cell Epulis)

Peripheral giant cell granuloma is not a true neoplasm but considered to be *a reactive lesion* due to local irritation or trauma (Fig. 11.12). Histologically, it *shows overlying mucosal surface composed of stratified squamous epithelium.* Sometimes it may show ulceration. The underlying *lesional tissue* consists of *multinucleated giant cells in a delicate fibrillar stroma* with ovoid or spindle-shaped fibroblasts. The *giant cells* are of varying size and may have only a few nuclei or more. Numerous capillaries are seen at the periphery of the lesion. *Foci of haemorrhage* with deposits of haemosiderin pigment is a *characteristic feature.* Acute and chronic inflammatory cell infiltrate is frequently present.

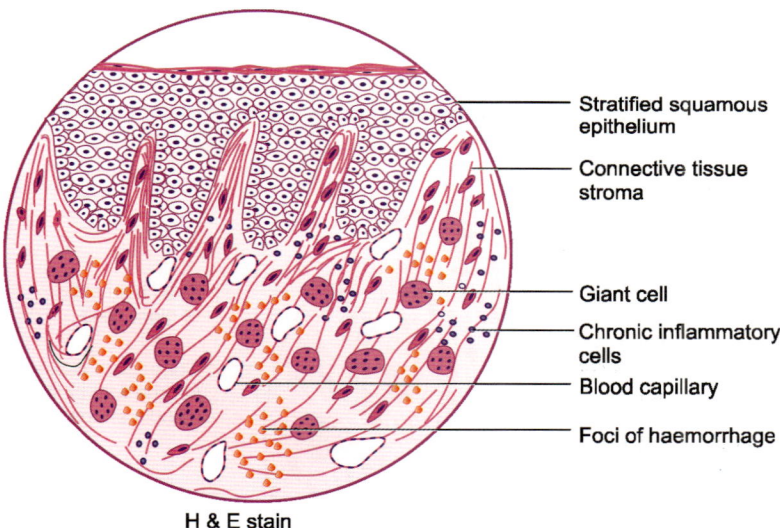

Stratified squamous epithelium

Connective tissue stroma

Giant cell

Chronic inflammatory cells

Blood capillary

Foci of haemorrhage

H & E stain

Figure 11.12 Peripheral giant cell granuloma — overlying stratified squamous epithelium and the underlying lesional tissue with scattered multinucleated giant cells and foci of haemorrhage.

Central Giant Cell Granuloma

Central giant cell granuloma is an *uncommon, benign* and *proliferative intraosseous lesion* of *unknown aetiology* (Fig. 11.13). It shows *proliferating connective tissue stroma with multinucleated giant cells.* The giant cells vary in size (small or large and round or irregular) with variable number of nuclei. These *giant cells* may be *diffusely present throughout the lesion* or *focally aggregated. Numerous foci of extravasated blood* and associated haemosiderin pigment are prominently seen. *Osteoid or bone formation* is *evident* within the lesion. The adjacent connective tissue stroma is loosely arranged with proliferating fibroblasts and small capillaries.

Giant Cell Tumour

Giant cell tumour is a rare but locally aggressive *bone tumour* (Fig. 11.14). Histologically, it shows *large multinucleated giant cells* that are *usually uniformly distributed* throughout the lesion. These

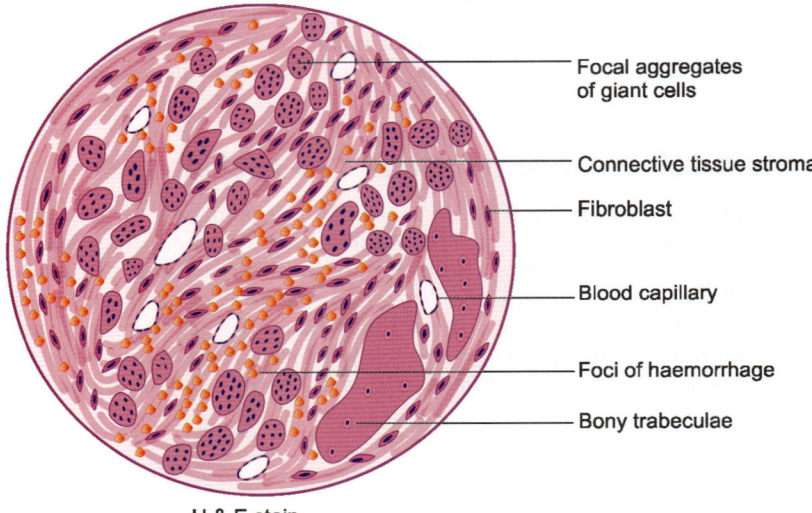

Focal aggregates
of giant cells

Connective tissue stroma

Fibroblast

Blood capillary

Foci of haemorrhage

Bony trabeculae

H & E stain

Figure 11.13   Central giant cell granuloma — proliferating connective tissue stroma with numerous multinucleated giant cells, foci of haemorrhage and bone formation.

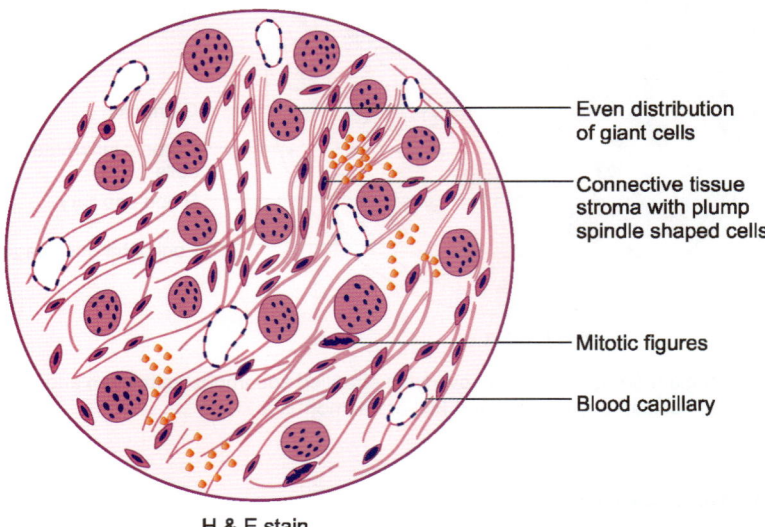

Even distribution
of giant cells

Connective tissue
stroma with plump
spindle shaped cells

Mitotic figures

Blood capillary

H & E stain

Figure 11.14   Giant cell tumour — large multinucleated giant cells in a connective tissue stroma with mitotic figures.

giant cells often contain as many as 40 to 60 nuclei. The *stromal cells* are *real tumour cells* and are mononuclear. They appear as uniform, plump, spindle-shaped or round-to-oval cells. Mitotic activity is commonly seen in the cellular connective tissue stroma. Areas of necrosis is a frequent feature.

Aneurysmal Bone Cyst

Aneurysmal bone cyst is a rare *benign intraosseous nonepithelial lined cystic lesion* of the craniofacial skeleton (Fig. 11.15). *Histologically,* it shows *blood-filled cystic spaces of variable sizes* in a *cellular*

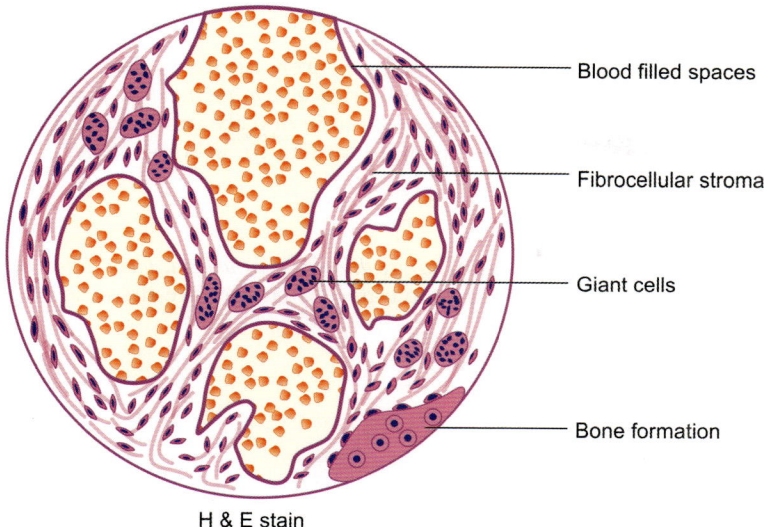

H & E stain

Figure 11.15   Aneurysmal bone cyst — blood-filled cystic spaces with no endothelial lining, cellular fibrous connective tissue stroma with multinucleated giant cells and trabeculae of bone.

fibrous connective tissue stroma. These *blood-filled spaces are not lined by endothelium. Multinucleated giant cells* are distributed within the connective tissue stroma. *Areas of haemosiderin deposits* are frequently seen. *Trabeculae of osteoid* or *woven bone* is also evident.

Lipoma

Lipoma is a *benign, slow growing* mesenchymal *neoplasm of mature fat cells* (Fig. 11.16). It occurs rarely in the oral cavity. *Histologically,* it is composed of *mature fat cells* surrounded by a thin fibrous capsule. When fibrous tissue is abundant, it is called fibrolipoma.

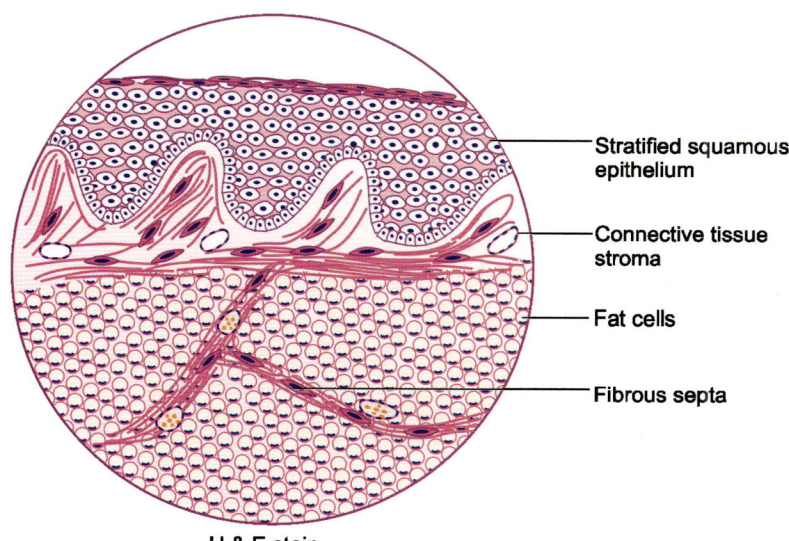

H & E stain

Figure 11.16   Lipoma — tumour composed of mature fat cells with fibrous septa within the lesion.

Capillary Haemangioma

Haemangiomas are *hamartomas of blood vessels* which rarely occur in the oral cavity (Fig. 11.17). *Histologically*, it is *composed of abundant small* capillaries *which are lined* by a *single layer of endothelial cells.* The adjacent connective tissue stroma is of variable density and resembles young granulation tissues. *Endothelial cell proliferation* may be a prominent feature in some cases.

Cavernous Haemangioma

The *cavernous haemangioma* is composed of *large, dilated, thin walled, blood filled vascular spaces with an endothelial lining* (Fig. 11.18). These are separated by connective tissue septa.

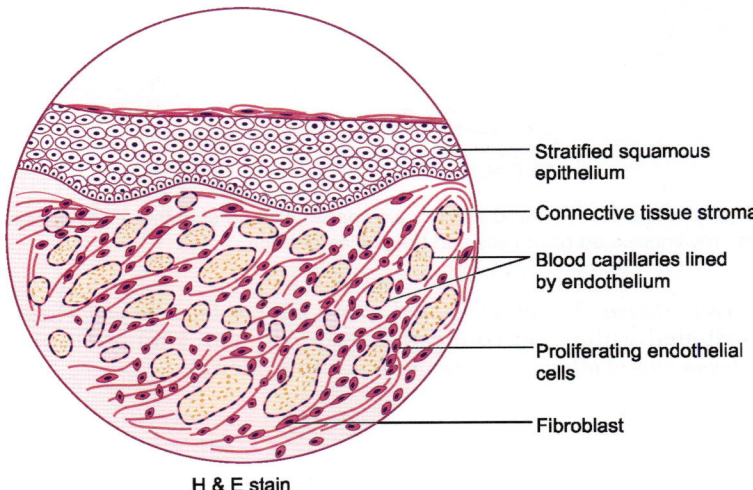

Stratified squamous epithelium

Connective tissue stroma

Blood capillaries lined by endothelium

Proliferating endothelial cells

Fibroblast

H & E stain

Figure 11.17   Capillary haemangioma — abundant small blood capillaries lined by endothelium and proliferation of endothelial cells.

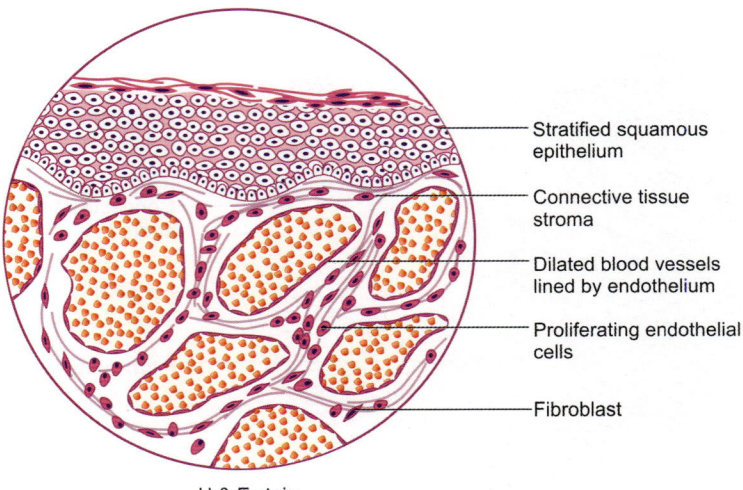

Stratified squamous epithelium

Connective tissue stroma

Dilated blood vessels lined by endothelium

Proliferating endothelial cells

Fibroblast

H & E stain

Figure 11.18   Cavernous haemangioma — large dilated blood vessels lined by endothelium.

Lymphangioma

The *lymphangiomas* are benign *hamartomatous lesions of* lymphatic *channels or vessels* (Fig. 11.19). In the oral cavity, it is located just below the overlying epithelium replacing the connective tissue papillae and *consists of multiple dilated* lymphatic *vessels* (cavernous type). These are *lined by a* single thin *layer of endothelial cells* and *contain lymph*. The adjacent connective tissue stroma is loose and fibrovascular.

Myxoma

Myxoma is a benign *neoplasm of mesenchyme-like* tissue *with abundant myxoid ground substance* (Fig. 11.20). Intraoral soft tissue myxoma is an extremely rare lesion. *Histologically*, it shows

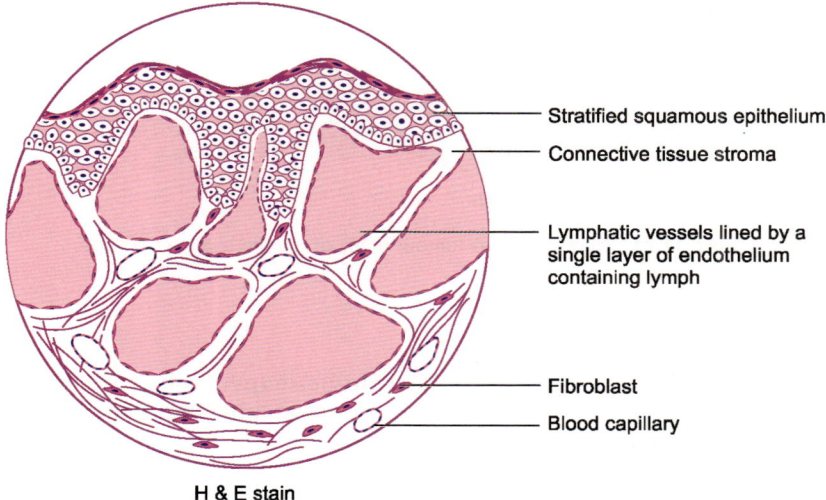

Stratified squamous epithelium

Connective tissue stroma

Lymphatic vessels lined by a single layer of endothelium containing lymph

Fibroblast

Blood capillary

H & E stain

Figure 11.19 Lymphangioma — multiple lymphatic vessels filled with lymph and lined by endothelium.

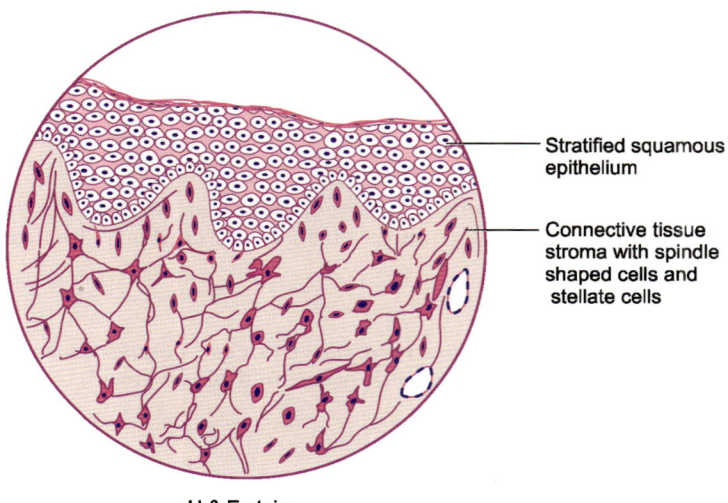

Stratified squamous epithelium

Connective tissue stroma with spindle shaped cells and stellate cells

H & E stain

Figure 11.20 Myxoma — stellate and spindle-shaped cells in loose myxoidstroma.

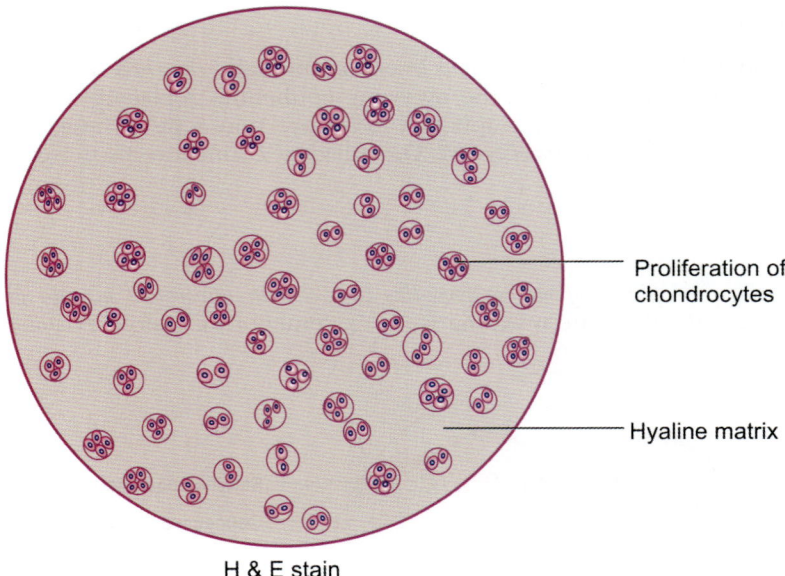

H & E stain

Figure 11.21   Chondroma — tumour mass of mature hyaline cartilage.

variable number of stellate cells and occasionally spindle-shaped cells with benign appearing nuclei. These tumour cells are embedded in a loose stroma having abundant myxoid or mucous background with reticulin fibres.

Chondroma

Chondroma is a *benign* intraosseous *tumour composed of* mature *hyaline cartilage* (Fig. 11.21). It is uncommon in the jaws. *Histologically,* it appears as a *circumscribed tumour mass* of *mature hyaline cartilage.* The small chondrocytes with pale cytoplasm and small, round nuclei within lacunae are evident. These tumour cells are benign without any malignant features. Areas of calcification or necrosis may be seen.

Osteoma

Osteoma is a *benign neoplasm* composed of *proliferation of compact* or *cancellous bone* in subperiosteal (peripheral) or occasionally endosteal (central) location (Fig. 11.22A and B).

Compact Osteoma

Compact osteoma is composed of *well-circumscribed mass* of dense *lamellar bone arranged like layers of an onion* with only *minimal marrow elements* (with occasional blood vessels and no Harversian system) (Fig. 11.22A).

Cancellous Osteoma

Cancellous osteoma is composed of *trabeculae of cancellous bone* with fibrofatty marrow spaces (Fig. 11.22B). *Osteoblastic activity may* be *seen.*

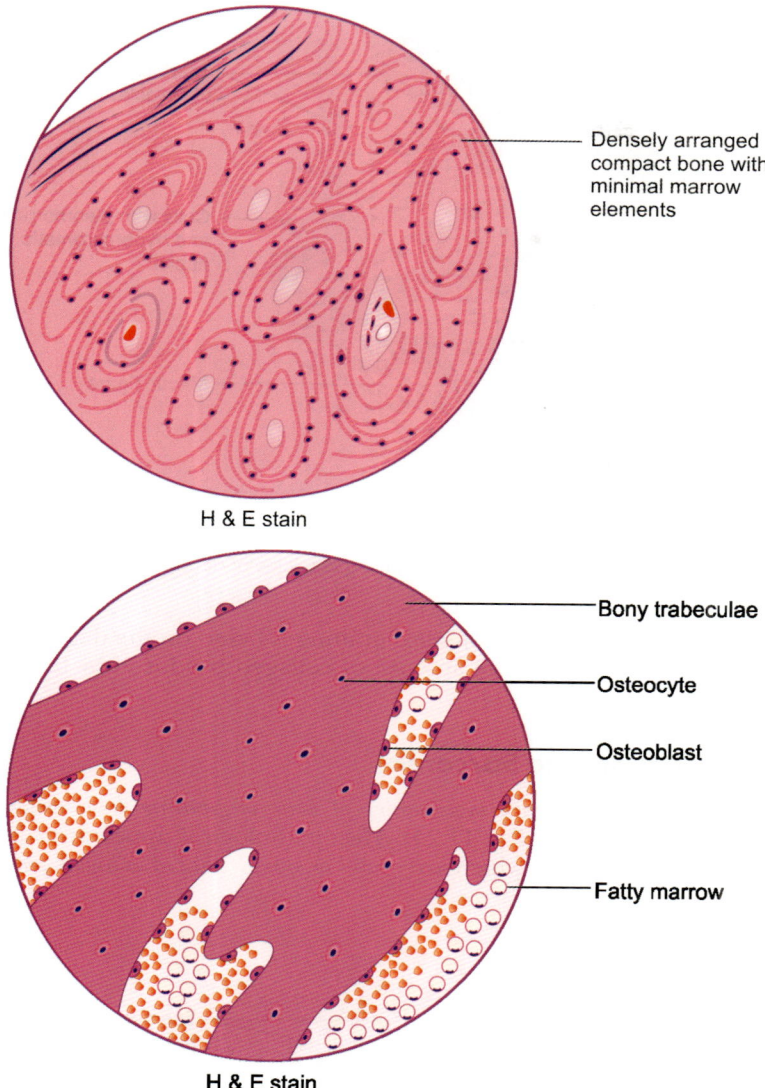

Densely arranged compact bone with minimal marrow elements

H & E stain

Bony trabeculae

Osteocyte

Osteoblast

Fatty marrow

H & E stain

Figure 11.22   (A) Osteoma (compact) – densely arranged compact bone with minimal marrow elements. (B) Osteoma (cancellous) – trabeculae of cancellous bone with osteoblastic activity.

MALIGNANT TUMOURS OF CONNECTIVE TISSUE ORIGIN

Fibrosarcoma

Fibrosarcoma is a malignant *neoplasm of fibroblasts* that rarely affects the oral cavity (Fig. 11.23). It may either arise in the soft tissue or be of primary intaosseous origin. It shows *proliferation of malignant fibroblasts* with variable amount of collagen and reticulin fibre formation. These cells are *spindle-shaped with* elongated, *oval, round hyperchromatic nuclei* with little variation in size and shape. The *tumour is cellular* and has typical *herringbone pattern*, i.e. interlacing fascicles of neoplastic

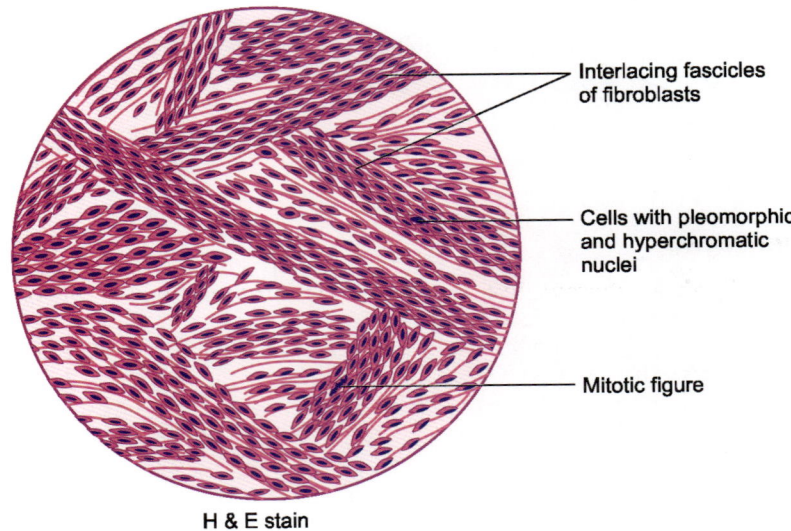

H & E stain

Figure 11.23 Fibrosarcoma — interlacing fascicles of neoplastic fibroblasts.

fibroblast. Mitotic figures are seen. Histological grading is based on the degree of cellularity, cellular differentiation, mitotic activity, the amount of collagen produced by tumour cells and the extent of necrosis.

Osteosarcoma (Osteogenic Sarcoma)

Osteosarcoma is the common *primary malignancy of bone originating from mesenchymal cells that are able to form bone or osteoid tissue* (Fig. 11.24). Histopathological appearance is highly variable. There is a *proliferation of tumour cells* which are *round or spindle shaped to highly pleomorphic cells* with

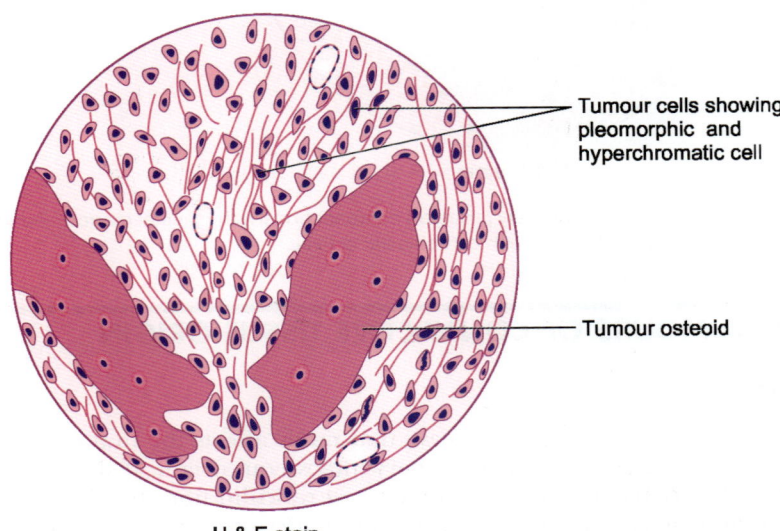

H & E stain

Figure 11.24 Osteosarcoma — proliferation of neoplastic cells and tumour osteoid.

considerable variation in size and shape. They may be small and angular or large and hyperchromatic. The *characteristic feature is the presence of osteoid formed by malignant osteoblasts* (tumour osteoid). The stromal cell may be osteoblastic, chondroblastic and/or fibroblastic without any prognostic significance.

BENIGN TUMOURS OF NERVE TISSUE ORIGIN

Traumatic Neuroma

Traumatic neuroma is an exuberant but nonneoplastic proliferation of nerve occurring in response to an injury or surgery (reactive hyperplasia of nerve tissue) (Fig. 11.25). Histologically, it shows haphazard proliferation of nerve fascicles including axons, Schwann cells and fibroblasts within a fibrous connective tissue stroma which may be dense or myxomatous in nature.

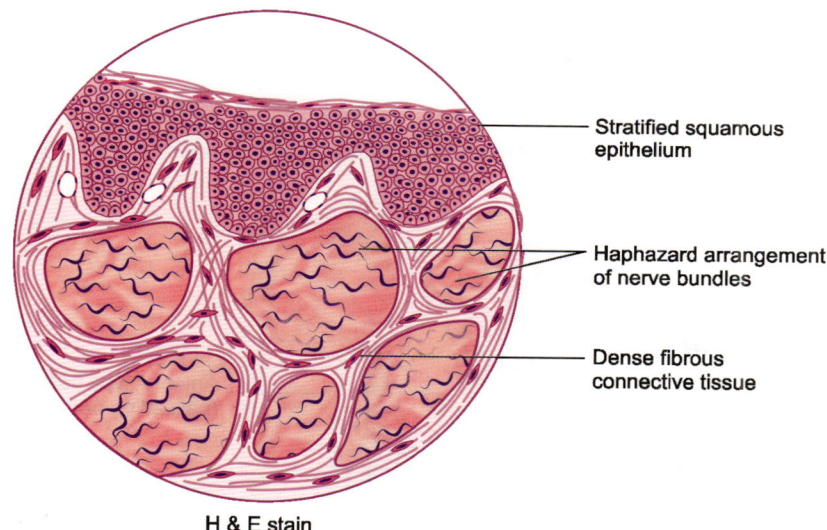

Stratified squamous epithelium

Haphazard arrangement of nerve bundles

Dense fibrous connective tissue

H & E stain

Figure 11.25 Traumatic neuroma — haphazard proliferation of nerve fascicles in a fibrous connective tissue stroma.

Neurofibroma

Neurofibroma is a *benign tumour of nerve tissue origin* and arises *from cells* that *constitute the nerve sheath* (i.e. mixture of cell type including Schwann cell and perineural fibroblasts) (Fig. 11.26). The *tumour is* composed of *cellular proliferation of delicate spindle-shaped cell* with *thin, wavy nuclei* arranged in a loose disorganized pattern. The connective tissue stroma consists of delicate collagen fibrils and variable amounts of myxoid matrix. Mast cells are often abundant.

Neurilemmoma (Schwannoma)

Neurilemmoma is a benign neural tumour that originates, from the Schwann cells of the neural sheath (Fig. 11.27). The microscopic picture is characteristic. It *consists of two types of tissues, Antoni type A tissue and Antoni type B tissue. Antoni type A* tissues usually *predominates* and *forms streaming fascicles of elongated spindle-shaped cells (Schwann cells),* nuclei of which are aligned in parallel rows forming a typical palisading pattern. *Antoni type B tissue is*

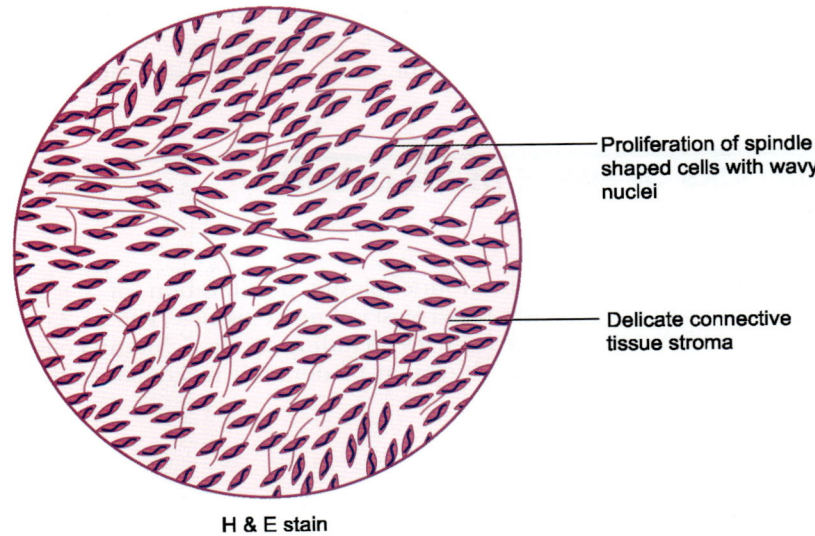

H & E stain

Figure 11.26 Neurofibroma — proliferation of spindle-shaped cells with thin and wavy nuclei.

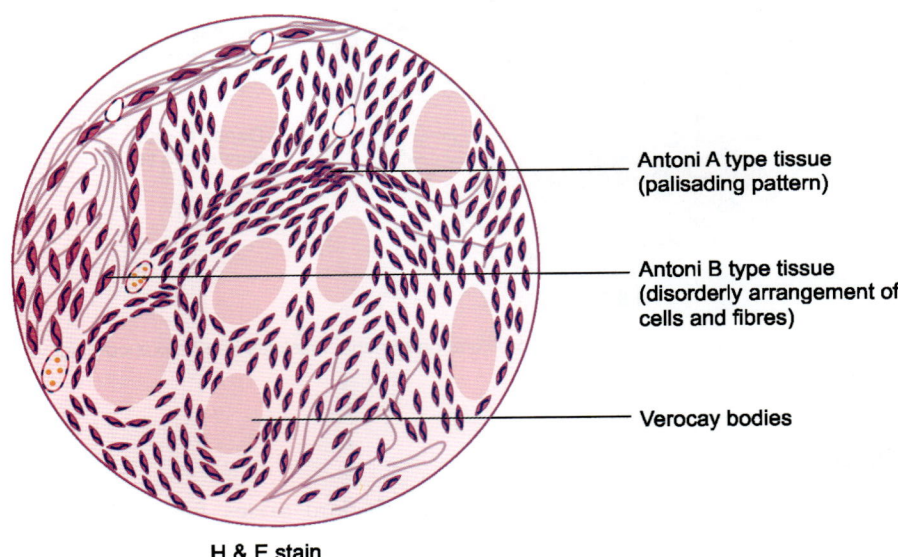

H & E stain

Figure 11.27 Neurilemmoma — well-circumscribed Antoni A tissue (palisading pattern) and Antoni B tissue (disorderly arranged) with verocay bodies (acellular eosinophilic masses).

less cellular and *consists of disorderly arrangement of elongated cells (spindle shaped)* and *fibres within a loose myxomatous stroma. Verocay bodies* which appear as *acellular, eosinophilic masses* are characteristically present in tumour. These are areas of reduplicated basement membrane and cytoplasmic processes.

Tumours of Salivary Glands | 12

PLEOMORPHIC ADENOMA (BENIGN MIXED TUMOUR)

Pleomorphic adenoma is the most *common benign salivary gland neoplasm* (Fig. 12.1). *Microscopic diversity is the characteristic feature* of this tumour. It is a *well-circumscribed* and encapsulated tumour with a capsule of variable thickness. The capsule may be incomplete or may show focal infiltration by the tumour cells. The tumour shows *glandular epithelium* and *myoepithelial cells* within a mesenchyme like tissue in a highly variable amount. The *epithelial component* may occur as *sheets, islands, cords or duct-like and small cyst-like structures of cells. Myoepithelial cells* are commonly seen with a *variable morphology* as *angular, spindle shaped or resembling plasma cells.* The

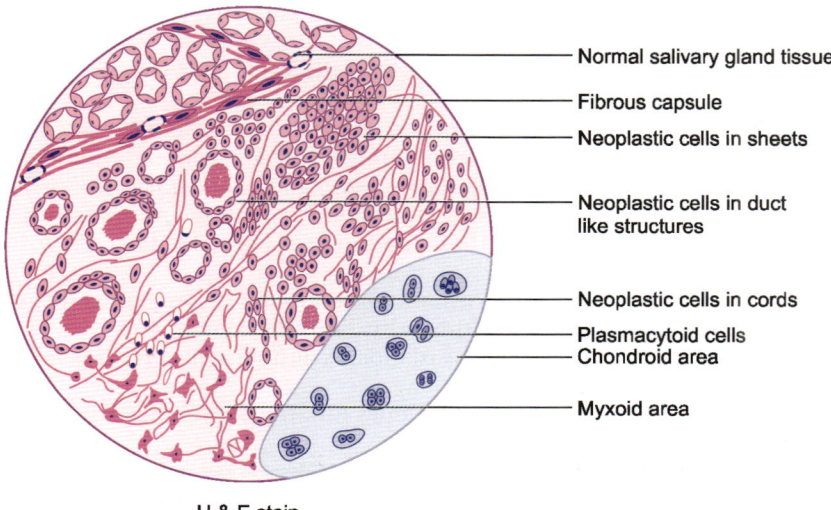

Normal salivary gland tissue

Fibrous capsule

Neoplastic cells in sheets

Neoplastic cells in duct like structures

Neoplastic cells in cords

Plasmacytoid cells

Chondroid area

Myxoid area

H & E stain

Figure 12.1 Pleomorphic adenoma — encapsulated tumour with neoplastic cells arranged in sheets, duct-like structures and cords and adjacent chondroid and myxoid areas.

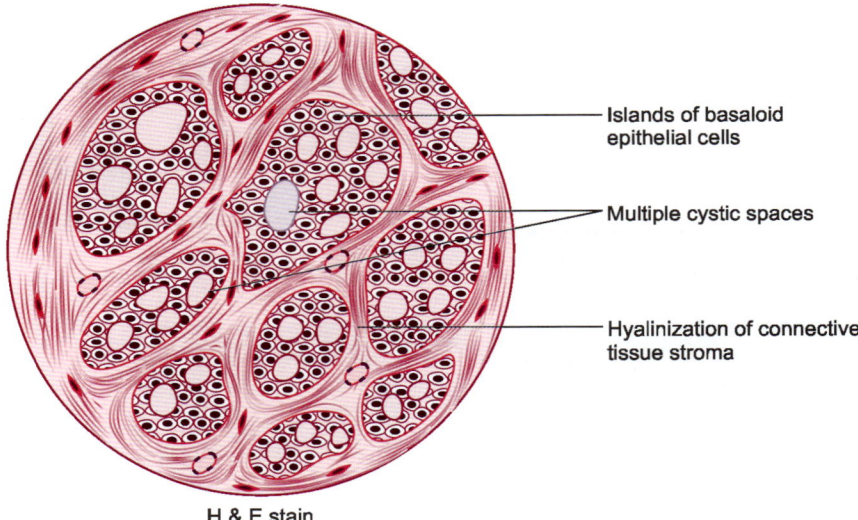

H & E stain

Figure 12.2   Adenoid cystic carcinoma — characteristic cribriform pattern showing multiple islands of basaloid cells and cyst-like spaces with the presence of basophilic mucoid material and hyalinization of connective tissue stroma.

characteristic stromal changes are due to pluripotential properties of myoepithelial cells so that *accumulations of mucoid material* resulting in the formation of *myxomatous areas, cartilaginous areas or eosinophilic hyalinized area.* Sometimes *osteoid* or fat cells are also seen. Squamous metaplasia is common.

ADENOID CYSTIC CARCINOMA

Adenoid cystic carcinoma is a malignant *tumour of the salivary glands* (Fig. 12.2). It is characterized by *proliferation of myoepithelial* cells and *ductal cells* in varied patterns: (i) *cribriform,* (ii) *tubular* and (iii) *solid.*

There may be a combination of these patterns and the tumour is classified according to the predominant pattern.

The *cribriform pattern* is the *characteristic pattern* and is *characterized by basaloid epithelial cells* (tumour cells) *arranged in the form of islands* or *nests,* containing *multiple cylindrical cyst-like spaces resembling Swiss cheese or honeycomb. The tumour cells are uniform, small* and *cuboidal with less cytoplasm* and *basophilic nuclei. The cyst-like spaces show presence of a hyalinized eosinophilic material, a basophilic mucoid material* or a *combination of both.* Sometimes these tumours cells forming the cribriform pattern are surrounded by hyalinized stroma.

In the tubular pattern, the tumour cells form multiple tubular or small duct-like structures that are lined by one to several layers of cells, within a hyalinized stroma.

The solid variant shows large solid sheets or islands of tumour cells with less tendency towards duct or cyst formation.

A characteristic feature of this tumour is its tendency towards perineural or intraneural invasion.

MUCOEPIDERMOID CARCINOMA

The *mucoepidermoid carcinoma* is one of the *most common malignant epithelial neoplasms of the salivary glands* (Fig. 12.3). As the name suggests, it consists of *mucous producing cells, epidermoid (squamous) cells and intermediate cells* (a third type of cells) *in varying proportions.*

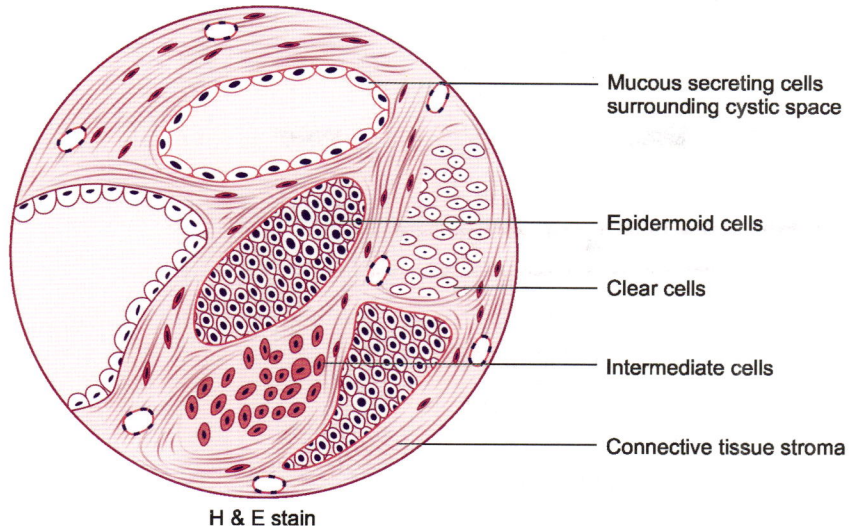

Mucous secreting cells surrounding cystic space

Epidermoid cells

Clear cells

Intermediate cells

Connective tissue stroma

H & E stain

Figure 12.3 Mucoepidermoid carcinoma – mucous-secreting cells surrounding a cystic space, sheets of epidermoid cells, intermediate cells and clear cells.

The *mucous cells are variable in shapes* with *abundant pale foamy cytoplasm lining* the cystic spaces as single or multiple layers. These cysts may rupture with liberation of mucus following inflammatory reaction. *These cells stain positively* with *mucin stains.* The *epidermoid cells are polygonal in shape* with intercellular bridges and found lining the cystic spaces with intermediate or mucous cells or may form solid islands. These cells rarely show keratinization. The *intermediate cells vary in appearance either from small, darkly staining basaloid cells to ovoid cells* with pale eosinophilic scanty cytoplasm. These cells are believed to be the progenitors of epidermoid and mucous cells. Variable number of clear cells can be present, which are generally glycogen and mucin free.

The tumour is graded as low grade, intermediate grade and high grade, depending on the amount of cyst formation, degree of cytologic atypia or the number of mucous, epidermoid and intermediate cells.

Odontogenic Cyst | 13

ODONTOGENIC KERATOCYST

Odontogenic keratocyst is a *developmental odontogenic epithelial lined cyst of the jaw*, with a biological behaviour similar to a benign neoplasm (Fig. 13.1). The histopathological features are characteristic. The *cystic lumen is* lined by a *stratified squamous epithelium of uniform thickness about 6–10 cells thick.* The *luminal surface layer* is *parakeratinized with wavy, corrugated or wrinkled appearance.* Sometimes it may be orthokeratinized with a prominent stratum granulosum. The *basal cell layer is well defined* and *composed of a prominent palisaded polarized layer of cuboidal or columnar cells* resembling *'picket fence'* or

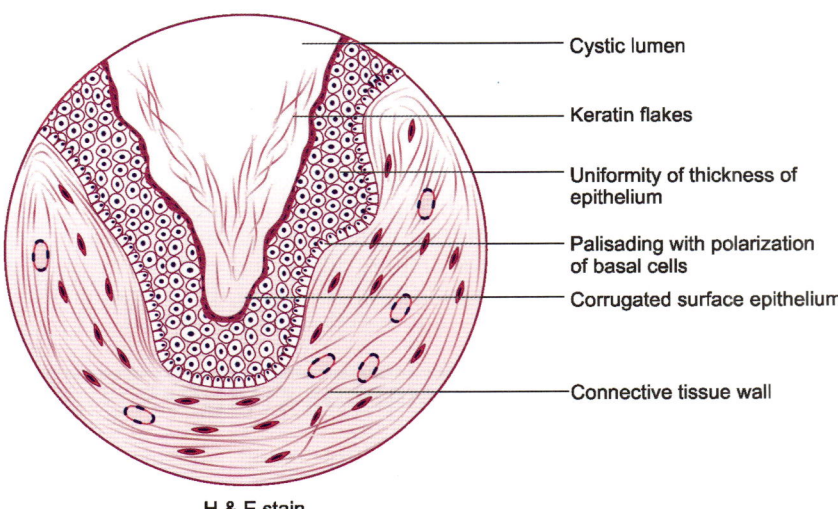

Cystic lumen

Keratin flakes

Uniformity of thickness of epithelium

Palisading with polarization of basal cells

Corrugated surface epithelium

Connective tissue wall

H & E stain

Figure 13.1 Odontogenic keratocyst — cystic lumen lined by parakeratinized corrugated surface with uniformity of thickness of epithelium and palisaded hyperchromatic basal cell layer.

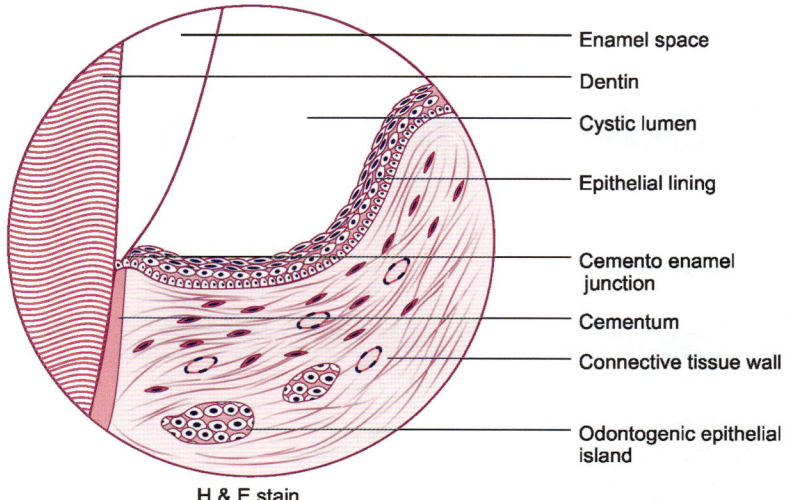

H & E stain

Figure 13.2   Dentigerous cyst — noninflammed dentigerous cyst with a cystic lumen lined by a thin nonkeratinized stratified sqamous epithelium lining attached to cementoenamel junction (CEJ) and the connective tissue wall with odontogenic epithelial islands.

'tombstone' appearance. The nuclei of the columnar basal cells in the parakeratinized lining are hyperchromatic and oriented away from the basement membrane. The *epithelium and connective tissue interface is usually flat* without rete ridges. The *connective tissue wall is thin,* fibrous and often shows *small satellite or daughter cysts, cords or islands of odontogenic epithelium.* The inflammatory cells are usually absent or scanty. In the presence of an intense inflammation, the epithelium may thicken and develop rete processes. The lumen may be filled with a clear fluid or cheesy material which consists of keratinous debris.

DENTIGEROUS CYST (FOLLICULAR CYST)

Dentigerous cyst is the *most common developmental odontogenic epithelial lined cyst* that *surrounds the crown of an unerupted tooth* and is *attached to the tooth at the cementoenamel junction* (Fig. 13.2). In the noninflamed dentigerous cyst, the epithelium lining consists of a thin layer of flattened nonkeratinized stratified squamous epithelium of about 2–4 cell layers. The epithelium and connective tissue interface is flat. The connective tissue wall is composed of a very loose fibrous connective tissue stroma and may show the presence of varying numbers of islands or cords of inactive odontogenic epithelium. In inflamed dentigerous cyst, the epithelial lining shows hyperplastic stratified squamous epithelium with development of rete ridges and variable chronic inflammatory cell infiltration. Rushton bodies within the lining epithelium are seen inflamed dentigerous cyst. The content of the cyst lumen is usually thin, watery-yellow fluid.

CYST UNDERGOING AMELOBLASTOMATOUS CHANGES

The dentigerous cyst might undergo neoplastic transformation and develop into *ameloblastoma* (Fig. 13.3).

Vickers and Gorlin criteria for this transformation when observed together are as follows:

1. Hyperchromatism of basal cell nuclei
2. Palisading with polarization of basal cells
3. Cytoplasmic vacuolization with intercellular spacing of lining epithelium

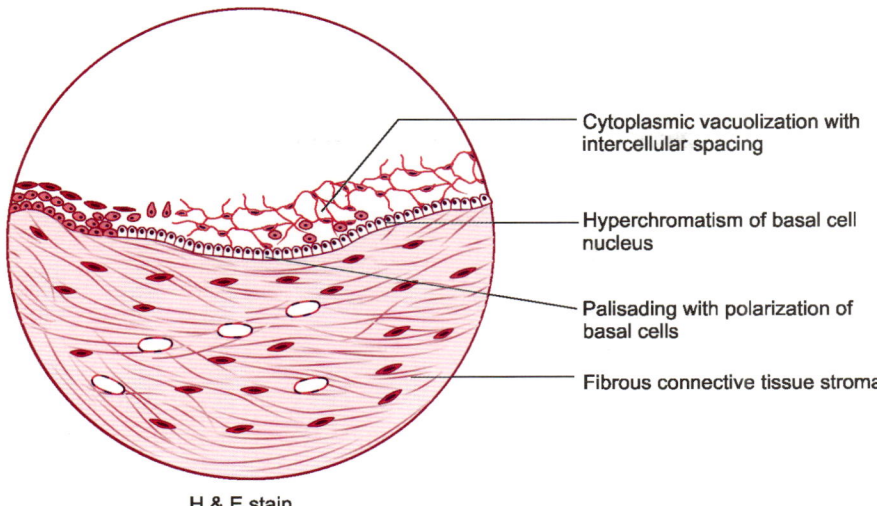

Cytoplasmic vacuolization with
intercellular spacing

Hyperchromatism of basal cell
nucleus

Palisading with polarization of
basal cells

Fibrous connective tissue stroma

H & E stain

Figure 13.3 Cyst undergoing ameloblastomatous changes.

CALCIFYING ODONTOGENIC CYST (GORLIN CYST)

Calcifying odontogenic cyst is an uncommon *developmental odontogenic* epithelial *lined cyst* (Fig. 13.4). The *cystic lumen* is lined by *odontogenic epithelium.* The basal *cell layer is cuboidal or columnar, resembling ameloblast-like cells* with an overlying loosely arranged stellate reticulum-like tissue. The most *characteristic feature* is the *presence of variable number of ghost cells within the epithelial lining.* These *ghost cells* are *altered epithelial cells* which are *larger in size* with *eosinophilic cytoplasm* and loss of nuclei with the preservation of basic cell outline. Masses of ghost cells may fuse to form large sheets of amorphous material. These *cells have affinity* to *undergo calcification.* Areas of *eosinophilic matrix* material resembling dysplastic dentin may be present adjacent to epithelial component. The connective *tissue wall is fibrocellular.*

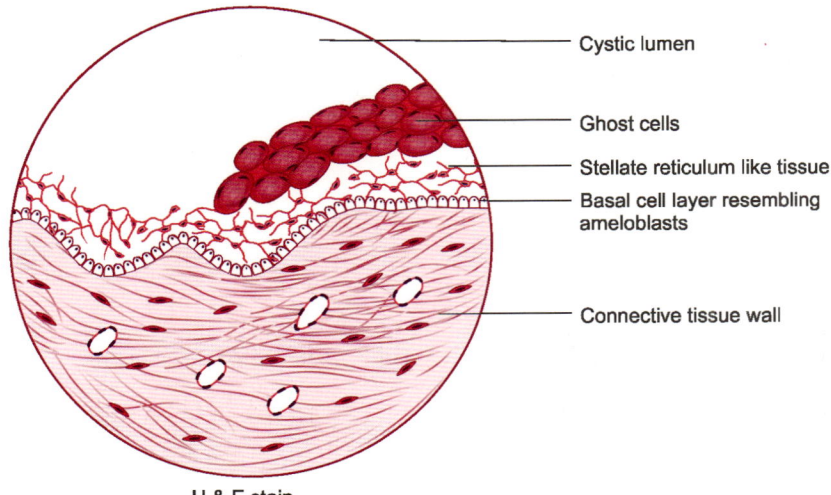

Cystic lumen

Ghost cells

Stellate reticulum like tissue

Basal cell layer resembling
ameloblasts

Connective tissue wall

H & E stain

Figure 13.4 Calcifying epithelial odontogenic cyst – cystic lumen lined by tall columnar basal cell layer with overlying stellate reticulum like tissue and ghost cells.

Odontogenic Tumours

AMELOBLASTOMA

Ameloblastoma is the *most common benign epithelial odontogenic tumour* without *odontogenic ectomesenchyme*. Histopathologic subtypes of ameloblastoma are as listed below.

Follicular Ameloblastoma

Follicular ameloblastoma is the *most common histopathologic pattern* (Fig. 14.1A). It consists of *many small discrete islands* of *epithelial cells* resembling *enamel organ epithelium* in a mature fibrous connective tissue stroma. These *epithelial islands consist* of a *peripheral layer of columnar or cuboidal cells* enclosing *a central core of polyhedral, loosely arranged cells* resembling *stellate reticulum.* The peripheral single layer (palisade) of tall columnar cells is similar to ameloblast-like cells with the nuclei at the opposite pole to the basement membrane (reversed nuclear polarity). In some areas, these peripheral cells may be cuboidal. *Cyst formation is common within the epithelial islands* due to degeneration of stellate reticulum-like cells. The adjacent connective tissue stroma is fibrocellular.

Plexiform Ameloblastoma

Plexiform ameloblastoma consists of *long, interconnecting strands or cords* of *odontogenic epithelium* (Fig. 14.1B). These strands are *bounded by columnar* or *cuboidal ameloblast-like cells* and *enclose the stellate reticulum-like cells* which are *less prominent.* Cyst formation is relatively uncommon and when occurs, it is due to the degeneration of connective tissue stroma rather than within the epithelium. The connective tissue stroma is loose and vascular.

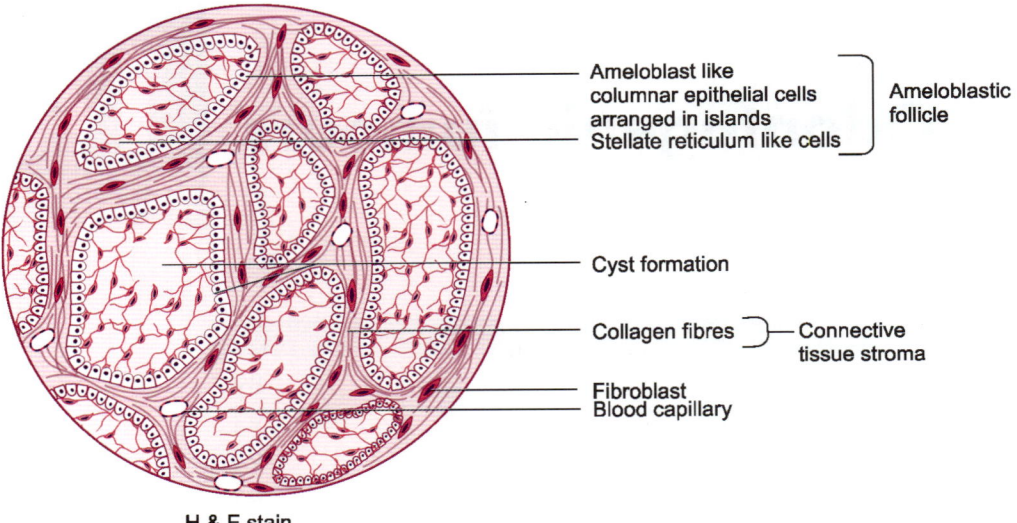

H & E stain

Figure 14.1A Follicular ameloblastoma — multiple islands of odontogenic epithelium with peripheral layer of columnar cells exhibiting reverse nuclear polarity and enclosing central core of stellate reticulum-like tissue which form the ameloblastic follicle. Cyst formation is common within these islands.

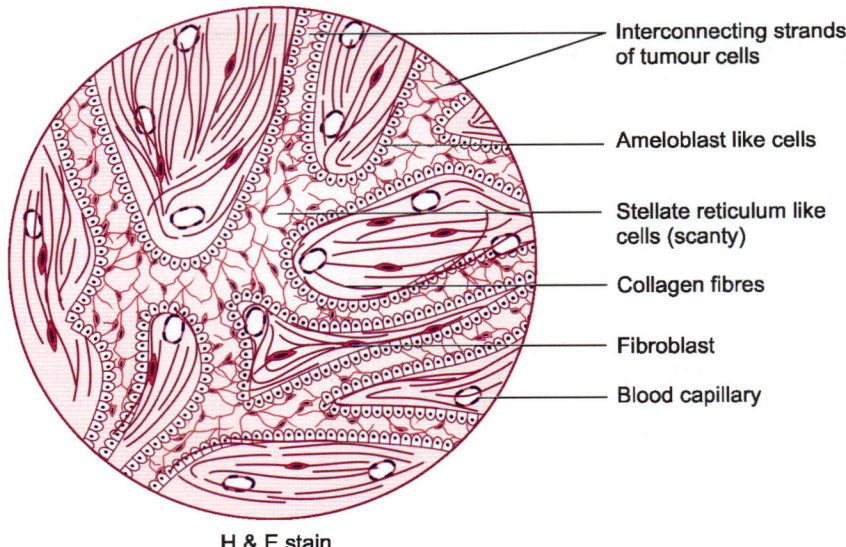

H & E stain

Figure 14.1B Plexiform ameloblatoma — interconnecting strands of odontogenic epithelium lined by cuboidal cells with less prominent (scanty) stellate reticulum-like tissue.

Acanthomatous Ameloblastoma

In *acanthomatous ameloblastoma*, the *central portion of epithelial islands* of a *follicular ameloblastoma resembling stellate reticulum-like tissue undergo squamous metaplasia* (Fig. 14.1C). Sometimes there may be keratin or epithelial pearl formation.

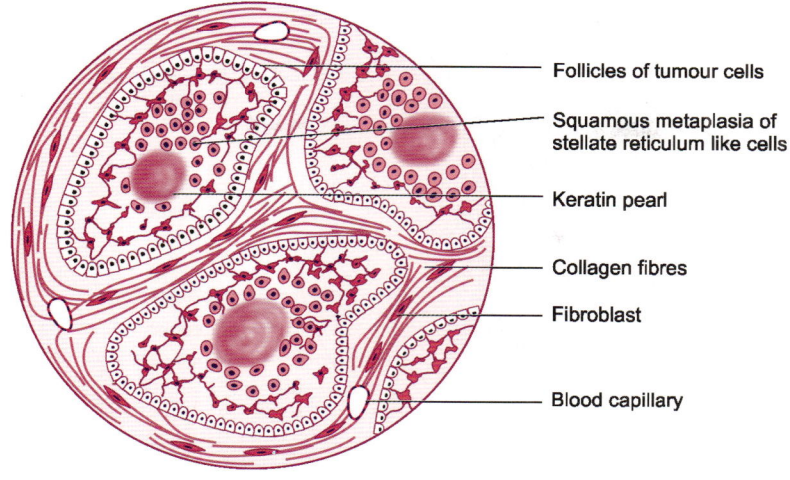

H & E stain

Figure 14.1C Acanthomatous ameloblastoma — follicles of ameloblastoma with squamous metaplasia of stellate reticulum-like tissue. Keratin pearl formation is also evident.

Granular Cell Ameloblastoma

In *granular cell ameloblastoma,* there is a *transformation of cytoplasm* of stellate *reticulum-like cells to granular cells* (Fig. 14.1D). These cells have abundant cytoplasm with *coarse eosinophilic granules* which are *lysosomal aggregates,* histochemically and ultrastructurally. This variant has been seen in young individuals and is considered to be *aggressive.*

Basal Cell Ameloblastoma

Basal cell ameloblastoma is the least *common type* and *resembles the basal cells carcinoma of skin* (Fig. 14.1E). It is *composed of nests of uniform basaloid cells with the peripheral cells cuboidal*

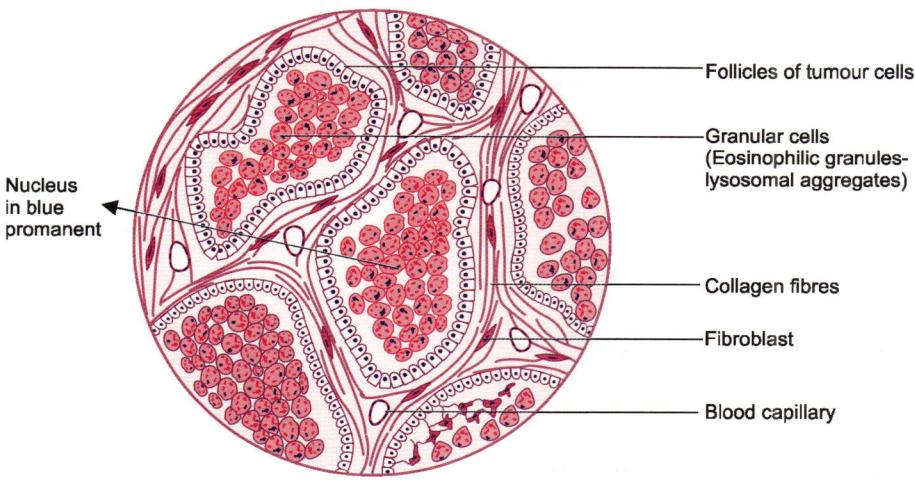

H & E stain

Figure 14.1D Granular cell ameloblastoma — follicles of ameloblastoma with transformation of cytoplasm of stellate reticulum-like cells to granular cells (central cell with prominent eosinophilic granular cytoplasm).

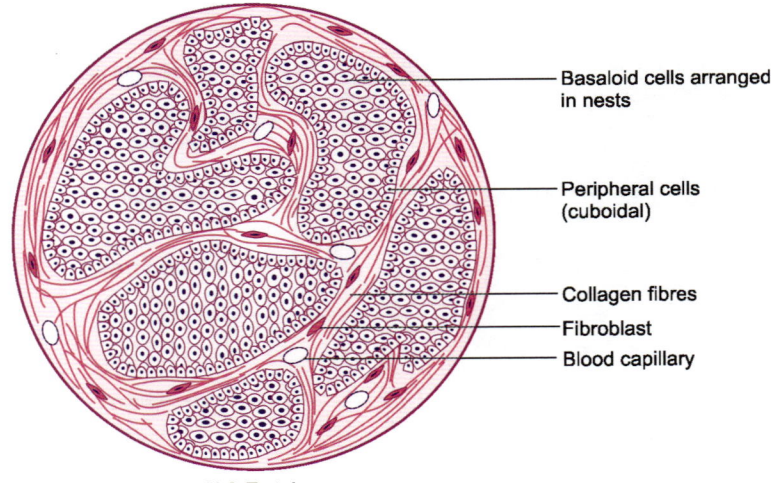

H & E stain

Figure 14.1E Basal cell ameloblastoma — islands of uniform, hyperchromatic basaloid cells with the peripheral cuboidal cells.

rather than columnar. There is no stellate reticulum-like tissue in the central portion of the nests.

Desmoplastic Ameloblastoma

Desmoplastic ameloblastoma bears little resemblance to the more common ameloblastoma (Fig. 14.1F). Characteristically, it shows a *dense collagenous stroma which is hyalinized* and *hypocellular.* The epithelial islands or cords are thin and seem to be compressed. The peripheral cells of these islands or cords are cuboidal or flattened instead of tall columnar. *Stellate reticulum-like tissue is also*

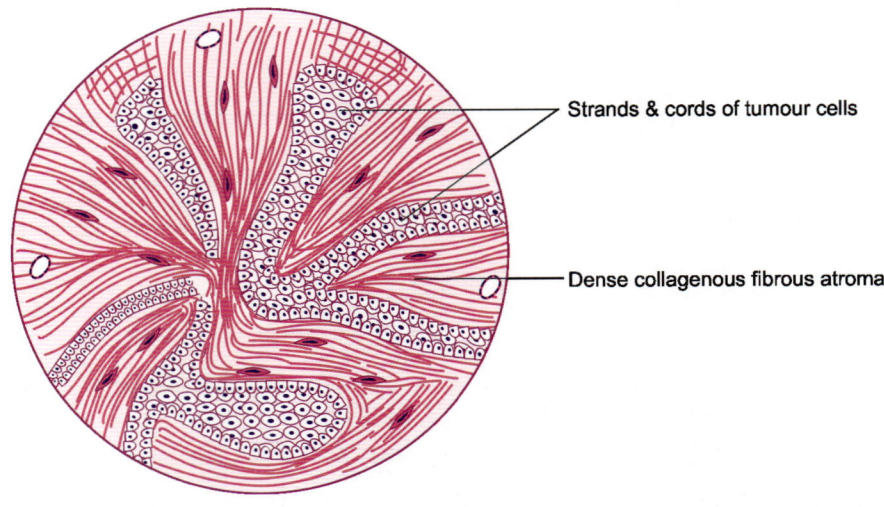

H & E stain

Figure 14.1F Desmoplastic ameloblastoma — dense hyalinized collagenous stroma with thin, compressed strands and chords of tumour cells (ameloblastic epithelium).

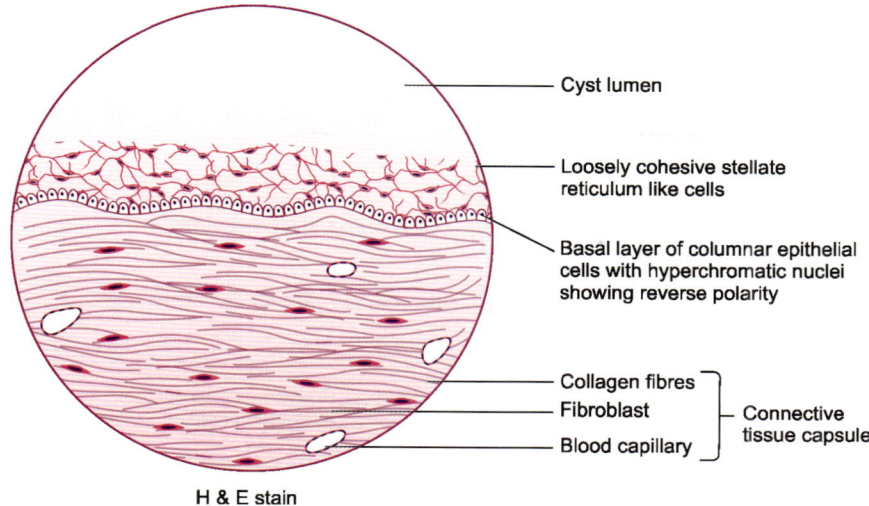

Cyst lumen

Loosely cohesive stellate reticulum like cells

Basal layer of columnar epithelial cells with hyperchromatic nuclei showing reverse polarity

Collagen fibres ⎫
Fibroblast   ⎬ Connective tissue capsule
Blood capillary ⎭

H & E stain

Figure 14.1G   Unicystic ameloblastoma (Luminal) — tumour confined to the luminal surface of the cyst with hyperchromatic, polarized columnar basal cell layer and overlying loosely arranged stellate reticulum-like tissue.

absent within this *epithelial islands* and show presence of *densely packed spindle-shaped or polygonal cells.* Calcification in the fibrous stroma and occasionally bone formation is seen.

Unicystic Ameloblastoma

Unicystic ameloblastoma is a variant of *ameloblastoma* (Fig. 14.1G). Histopathologically it is a cystic lesion that shows three groups:

(i) Typical *ameloblastomatous epithelial lining* of the *cyst cavity totally* and *partially;* and the *tumour is confined to* the luminal *surface of the cyst.* It shows columnar or cuboidal basal cell layer with hyperchromatic nuclei, reversal polarity and basilar cytoplasmic vacuolization – *luminal unicystic ameloblastoma.*

(ii) Nodular *proliferation of plexiform ameloblastoma* projecting *into the cystic lumen* without infiltration into the connective tissue wall – *intraluminal unicystic ameloblastoma.*

(iii) The fibrous cyst wall shows typical follicular or plexiform ameloblastoma of variable extent and depth – *mural unicystic ameloblastoma.*

CALCIFYING EPITHELIAL ODONTOGENIC TUMOUR (PINDBORG TUMOUR)

Calcifying epithelial odontogenic tumour also known as *Pindborg tumour* is a rare *benign epithelial odontogenic tumour* (Fig. 14.2). It has *variable appearances* but *typically shows islands, strands or sheets of polyhedral neoplastic epithelial cells* in a fibrous connective tissue stroma. These cells have a well-defined border with abundant eosinophilic finely granular cytoplasm and with nuclear pleomorphism and prominent nucleoli. The intercellular bridges are prominent. *Areas of an extracellular amorphous, eosinophilic hyalinized material (amyloid like)* are present. *Calcifications in the form of concentric rings (Liesegang rings)* develop within the amyloid-like material and may form large masses. A clear cell variant of this neoplasm exhibits the tumour cells with a clear vacuolated cytoplasm rather than an eosinophilic cytoplasm.

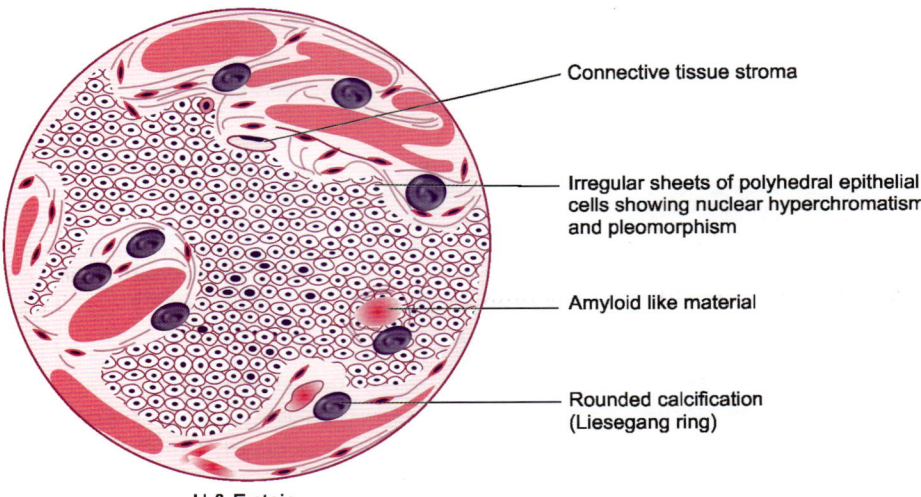

H & E stain

Figure 14.2 Calcifying epithelial odontogenic tumour — sheets of polyhdral neoplastic epithelial cells with eosinophilic cytoplasm and nuclear hyperchromatism and pleomorphism. Extracellular eosinophilic amyloid-like material and rounded calcifications (Liesegang rings) are seen.

ADENOMATOID ODONTOGENIC TUMOUR

Adenomatoid odontogenic tumour is considered to be an *uncommon benign epithelial odontogenic tumour* (Fig. 14.3). It is categorized as a hamartomatous lesion by some investigators. Histologically it has *well-defined, thick fibrous capsule*. The tumour is composed of *multinodular proliferation of cuboidal, columnar or spindle-shaped epithelial cells* in various patterns like *ductal or tubular structures, sheets, strands, whorled masses or rosette-like structures*. The duct-like or tubular structures are characteristic feature and consist of central lumen/space lined by a single layer of columnar or cuboidal epithelial

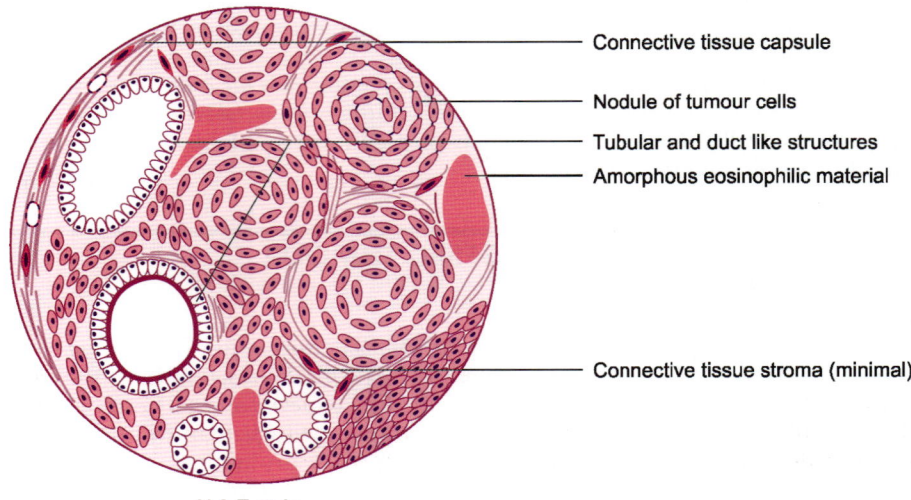

H & E stain

Figure 14.3 Adenomatoid odontogenic tumour — encapsulated tumour with epithelial tumour cells arranged in the form of nodules, tubular and duct-like structures. The nuclei of the cells in tubular and duct-like structures are away from the lumen. Amorphous eosinophilic material is seen.

cells nuclei of which are oriented away from the central lumen/space. The central space may be empty or contain small amounts of *eosinophilic material which may be* stained by *amyloid stain.* Spindle-shaped or polygonal closely opposed epithelial cells fill the spaces between these nodules. *Small foci of calcified bodies may be seen.* This has been considered as areas of abortive enamel formation, dentinoid or cementum. The connective tissue stroma is minimal.

AMELOBLASTIC FIBROMA

Ameloblastic fibroma is a true *mixed odontogenic tumour* in which there is a *proliferation of epithelial and mesenchymal components* without formation of enamel or dentin (Fig. 14.4). The *epithelial component* consists of *long, narrow interlacing, strands, cords or nests* of *proliferating odontogenic epithelium.* These epithelial cells are cuboidal and columnar and *resemble the dental lamina* of early tooth development. The stellate reticulum-like tissue is not always seen within these strands or sometimes the islands may enclose the loosely arranged stellate reticulum-like tissue. *The mesenchymal component consists of* plump stellate or ovoid cells in loose matrix with intertwining fibrils *resembling dental papilla.* Juxta-epithelial hyalinization is sometimes seen in the mesenchymal portion of the tumour.

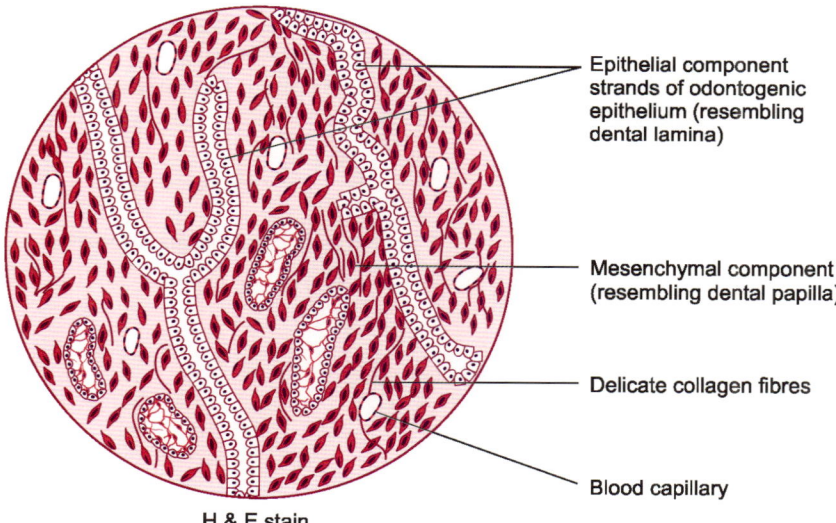

Epithelial component strands of odontogenic epithelium (resembling dental lamina)

Mesenchymal component (resembling dental papilla)

Delicate collagen fibres

Blood capillary

H & E stain

Figure 14.4   Ameloblastic fibroma — epithelial component composed of strands of odontogenic epithelium resembling dental lamina and mesenchymal component composed of highly cellular connective tissue stroma resembling dental papilla.

ODONTOMAS

Odontomas are the most *common types of mixed odontogenic tumours* and considered to be *hamartomas.* In this, both the *epithelial and mesenchymal cells* undergo *complete differentiation* so that the functional ameloblasts and odontoblasts *form enamel and dentin.* The lesion is *composed of more than* one type of *tissue,* so called as a *composite odontoma.*

Compound Composite Odontoma

Compound composite odontoma is composed of multiple, small, single rooted tooth-like structures in a loose fibrous *connective tissue stroma* (Fig 14. 5A). The enamel and dentin are laid down in a more

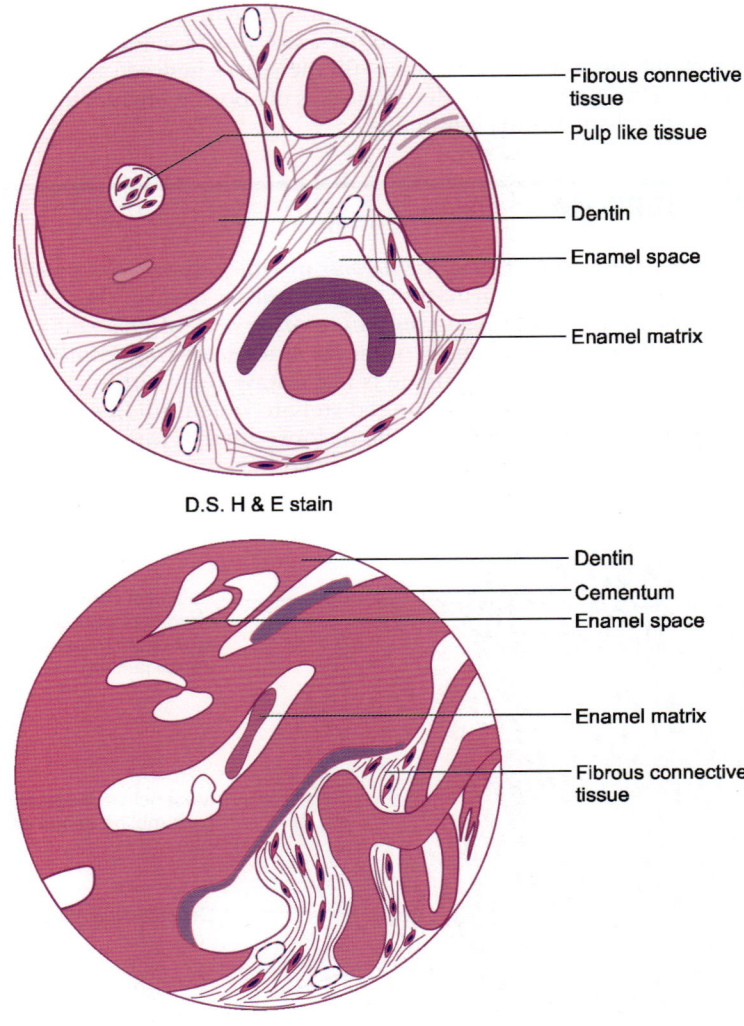

D.S. H & E stain

- Fibrous connective tissue
- Pulp like tissue
- Dentin
- Enamel space
- Enamel matrix

- Dentin
- Cementum
- Enamel space
- Enamel matrix
- Fibrous connective tissue

D.S. H & E stain

Figure 14.5 Odontoma: (A) compound odontoma — multiple tooth-like structures in a fibrous connective tissue stroma and (B) complex odontoma — hard and soft dental tissues with no morphological similarity to normal tooth.

orderly pattern so that there is a considerable resemblance to normal teeth. The mature enamel of these tooth-like structures are lost during the preparation of a microscopic section and appear as a clear space. Varying amounts of enamel matrix may be present. Pulp tissue is often seen within these tooth-like structures.

Complex Composite Odontoma

Complex composite odontoma consists of an *irregular mass of hard and soft dental tissues with no morphological similarity to normal teeth* (Fig. 14.5B). It shows large areas of mature tubular dentin. There are areas of mature enamel which are lost during microscopic preparation of section, enamel matrix or immature enamel and the thin layer of cementum at the periphery of the mass. Small foci of eosinophilic staining ghost cells may be seen rarely.

Regressive Alterations of Teeth

15

ATTRITION

Attrition is a physiologic wearing *away of tooth* as a result of *tooth- to- tooth contact* as in *mastication* (Fig. 15.1). It is seen on the *occlusal, incisal and proximal surfaces of the teeth*. There is *flattening of occlusal surfaces* with subsequent exposure of dentin. This results in the *formation* of *dead tracts and*

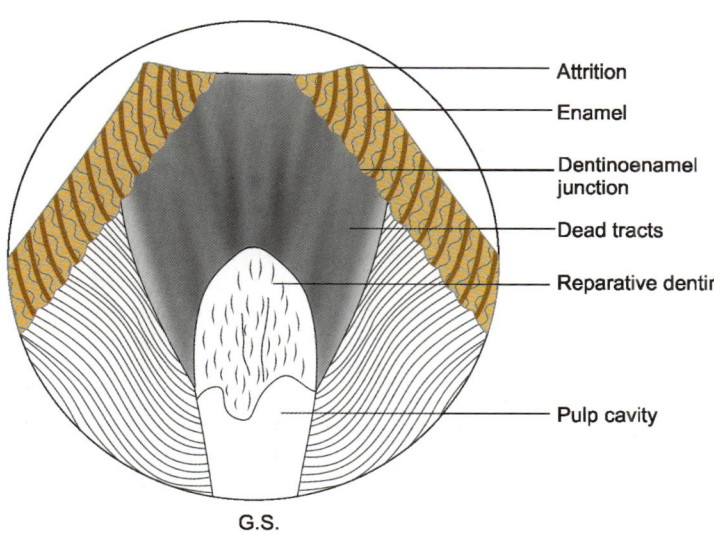

G.S.

Figure 15.1 Attrition (GS) — flattening of occlusal surface with formation of dead tracts and reparative dentin.

97

reparative dentin. Dead tracts are the areas characterized by degenerated odontoblastic processes which appear black in transmitted light and white in reflected light. Reparative dentin is formed as a response to attrition, often showing few and twisted dentinal tubules than normal dentin.

ABRASION

Abrasion is a *pathologic* wearing *away of tooth structure by abnormal mechanical forces* (Fig. 15.2). It *usually occurs at the cervical margins* on the *facial surfaces of the teeth* as a *result of faulty tooth brushing.* Incisal edges of anterior teeth may show V-shaped notching due to habitual opening of bobby pins with the teeth. This type of notching may also be seen in tailors, carpenters or shoemakers as a result of occupational hazard. The improper use of dental floss or toothpaste can be a form of abrasion on the proximal exposed root surfaces. There is formation of dead tracts and reparative dentin as a response to this pathologic process.

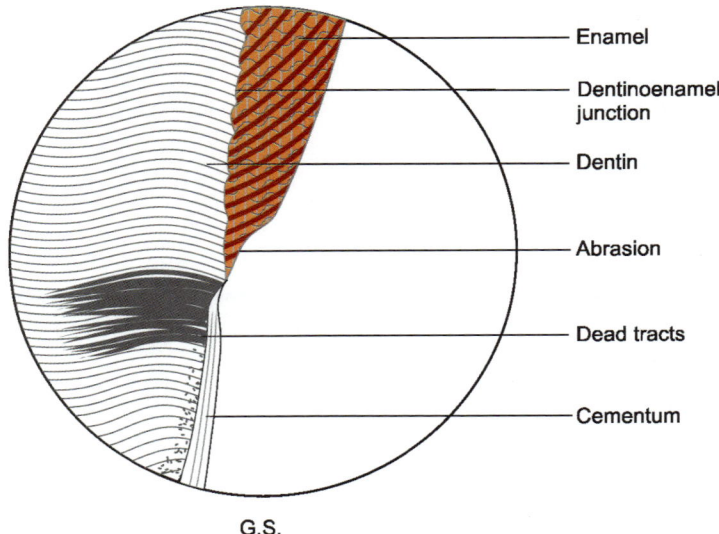

Enamel

Dentinoenamel junction

Dentin

Abrasion

Dead tracts

Cementum

G.S.

Figure 15.2   Abrasion (GS) — abrasion of cervical margin.

PULP FIBROSIS

Pulp fibrosis is a regressive *change in aging pulp* (Fig. 15.3). Pulp shows the *deposition of bundles of collagen fibres* and diffused fibrillar components. The *fibres are arranged more diffusely* in coronal pulp and longitudinally in radicular pulp. It is a gradual phenomenon and may occur as a result of any external trauma such as dental caries or deep restorations. It may also be due to increase in collagen in the medial and adventitial layers of blood vessels.

PULP STONES (DENTICLES) TRUE

Pulp stones are *nodular, mineralized structures* seen in *coronal and/or radicular pulp tissue* (Fig. 15.4).
    True pulp stones are rare and commonly *seen close to apical foramen.* These are formed by *odontoblasts* and resemble *secondary dentin in structure,* i.e. few and irregular dentinal tubules and odontoblasts on their surface. They may occur in functional and unerupted teeth. These may be

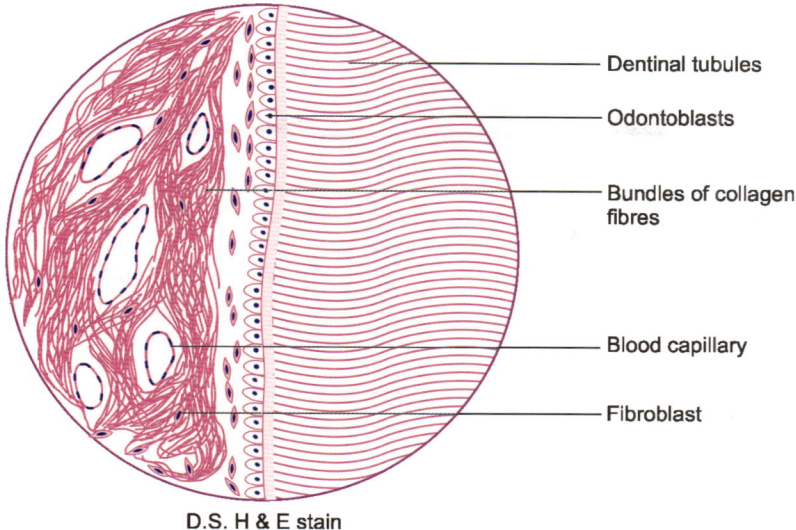

Dentinal tubules

Odontoblasts

Bundles of collagen fibres

Blood capillary

Fibroblast

D.S. H & E stain

Figure 15.3 Pulp fibrosis — deposition of dense collagen fibre bundles.

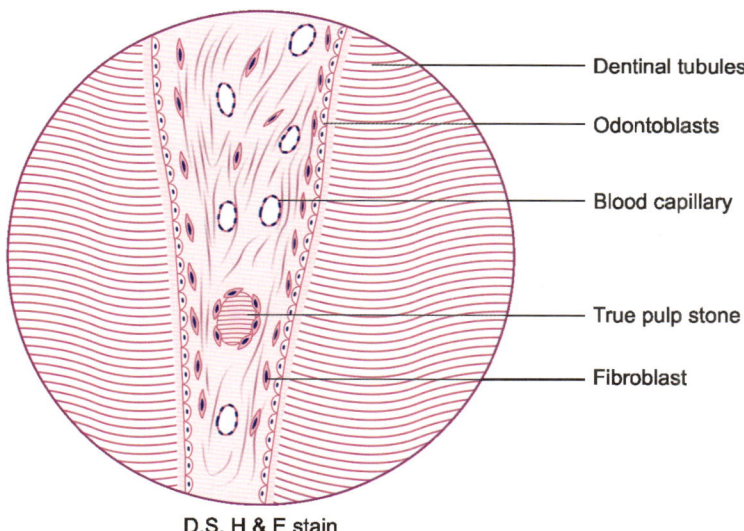

Dentinal tubules

Odontoblasts

Blood capillary

True pulp stone

Fibroblast

D.S. H & E stain

Figure 15.4 True pulp stones — true pulp stone which resembles the dentin and odontoblasts are seen on the surface.

subdivided as *free, attached or embedded,* depending *on their association with dentin.* Free pulp stones are completely surrounded by pulp tissue, attached pulp stones are partly fused to dentin and embedded pulp stones are completely surrounded by dentin.

PULP STONES (DENTICLES) FALSE

False pulp stones appear as *concentric layers of calcified tissue* (Fig. 15.5). These are *more common in pulp chambers as compared* to root canals. They *do not show the presence of dentinal tubules.* There is a central nidus around which calcification is seen *in the form of concentric layers.* It may be remnants of

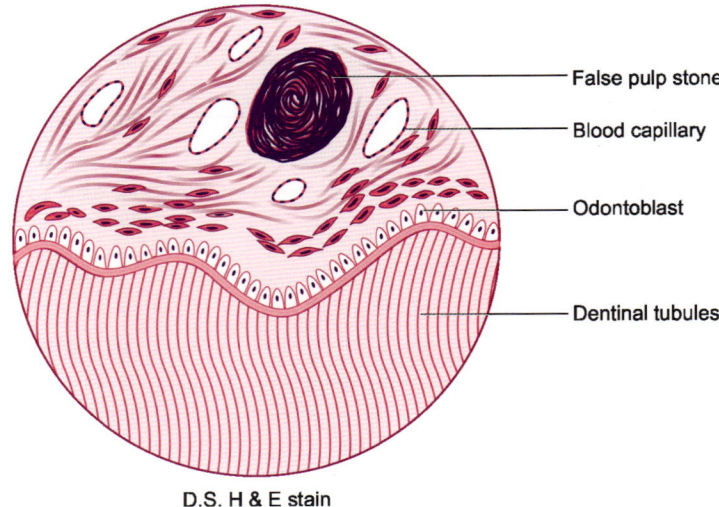

D.S. H & E stain

Figure 15.5 False pulp stones — false pulp stone as concentric layers of calcified tissue.

necrotic or calcified cells, calcification of thrombi of blood vessels (phleboliths) or calcification within a collagen fibre bundle. They may be *subdivided as free, attached or embedded depending on their association with dentin.*

DIFFUSE CALCIFICATIONS

Diffuse calcifications are *amorphous dystrophic calcifications* which appear as *irregular linear strands of calcific deposits* (Fig. 15.6). They are most commonly *seen in radicular pulp* and *supposed to be an age-related degenerative change.* They usually follow collagen fibre bundles or blood vessels.

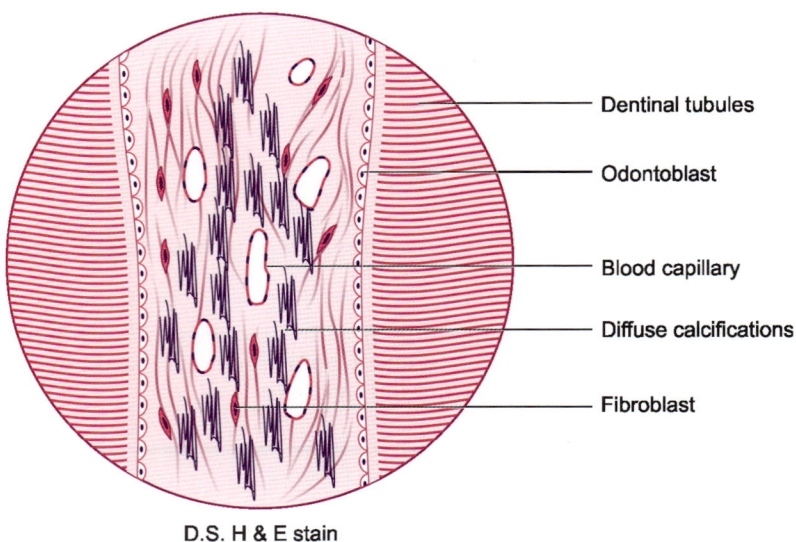

D.S. H & E stain

Figure 15.6 Diffuse calcifications — as irregular linear strands of calcific deposits.

HYPERCEMENTOSIS (CEMENTUM HYPERPLASIA)

Hypercementosis is considered as a *regressive change of tooth* but can also be a *pathological phenomenon* (Fig. 15.7). There is *deposition of excessive amount of cellular or secondary cementum on root surface.* It may be localized or diffuse, and may affect a single tooth or all the teeth or only part of one tooth. This cementum is arranged in the form of concentric layer around the root. *Accelerated elongation of tooth, inflammation about a tooth,* tooth repair and Generalized hypercementosis is seen in Paget's disease.

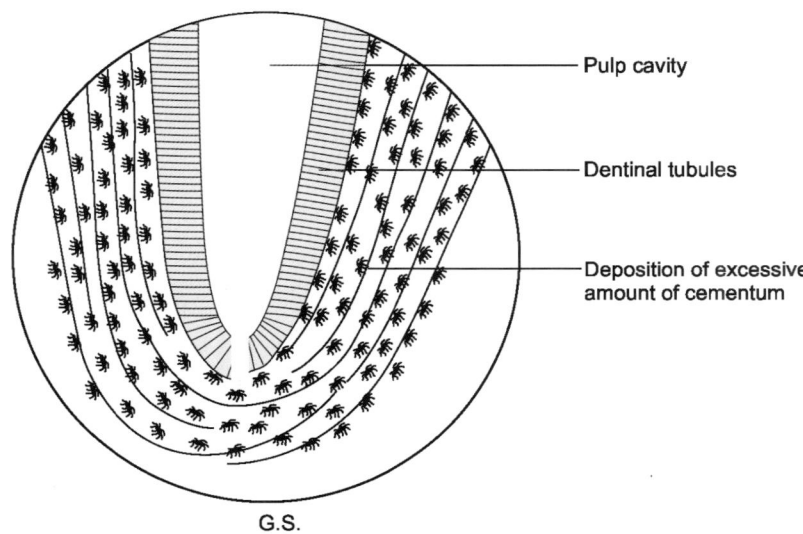

Pulp cavity

Dentinal tubules

Deposition of excessive amount of cementum

G.S.

Figure 15.7 Hypercementosis (GS) — deposition of excessive amount of cementum.

Bacterial and Mycotic Infections

16

STREPTOCOCCI

Streptococci are Gram-positive ovoid or *spherical cocci arranged in chains* (Fig. 16.1). These are part of the normal flora of human, inhabiting at various sites like mouth, skin, intestine and upper respiratory tract. There are *different types of streptococci, some of which are pathogenic.* The *infections vary in severity* from *mild throat infections to life-threatening infections.* Most streptococcal infections can be treated with antibiotics.

STAPHYLOCOCCI

Staphylococci are Gram-positive spherical *cocci arranged in grape-like clusters* (Fig. 16.2). These are frequent isolates from the oral cavity. These are the *commonest cause of suppuration* and are *responsible* for a *variety* of *common and uncommon infections.* Appropriate antibiotics should be given to treat these infections since drug resistance is common among staphylococci.

MYCOBACTERIUM TUBERCULOSIS

M. tuberculosis is a pathogenic acid-fast bacilli and the *causative agent of tuberculosis* (Fig. 16.3). It is a *slender, straight* or slightly *curved bacillus occurring singly, in pairs* or in small clumps. *Ziehl–Neelsen stain* (acid-fast stain) is useful to *stain these bacilli,* where these are seen as bright-red bacilli and tissue cells, and other organisms seen as blue.

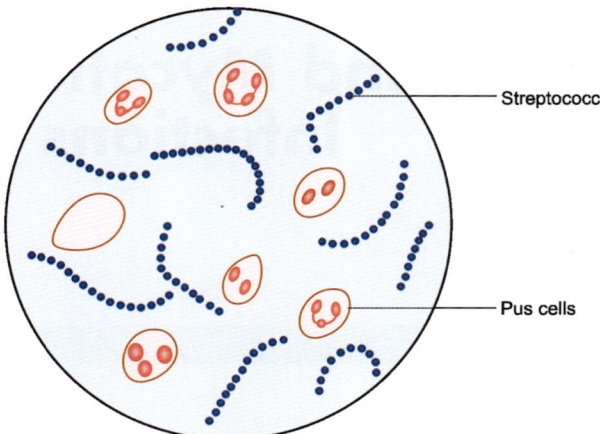

Figure 16.1 Streptococci — Gram-positive cocci in chains.

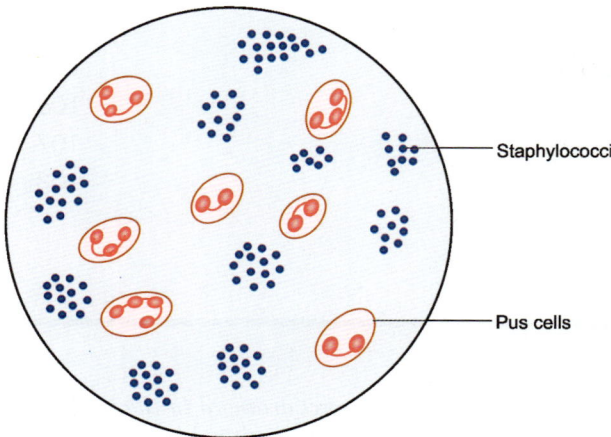

Figure 16.2 Staphylococci — Gram-positive cocci in clusters.

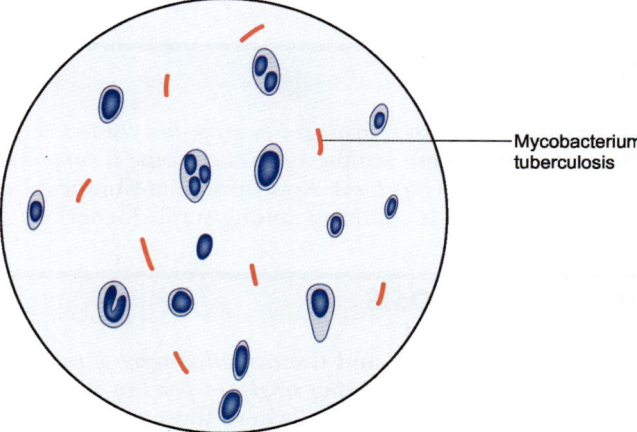

Figure 16.3 *Mycobacterium tuberculosis* — slender, acid-fast bacilli (bright red in colour).

TUBERCULOUS GRANULOMA

Tuberculous granuloma is an immune response to M. tuberculosis (Fig. 16.4). *It is a circumscribed area of infection,* often with central *caseous necrosis surrounded* by *epithelioid histiocytes, lymphocytes* and *multinucleated giant cells* also known as *Langhans giant cells.* Langhans *giant cells are large, multinucleated, oval-to-round* cells with *nuclei arranged either around the periphery in the form of horseshoe or ring or* clustred at the two poles of the giant cell.

MYCOBACTERIUM LEPRAE

M. leprae is the *causative agent of a chronic infectious disease,* i.e. *leprosy* (Hansen disease). It is a *straight* or *slightly curved rod-shaped bacillus* with considerable morphological variation (Fig. 16.5). It is *stained with Ziehl–Neelsen (acid-fast stain).* The bacilli may occur singly or in groups

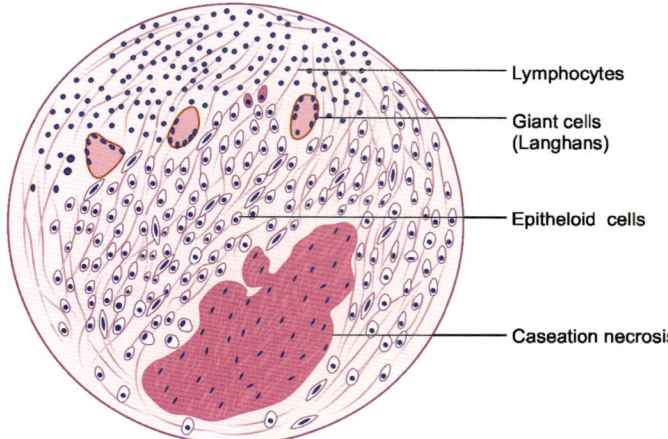

Figure 16.4 Tuberculous granuloma — caseous necrosis, epitheloid histocytes, lymphocytes and Langhans giant cells.

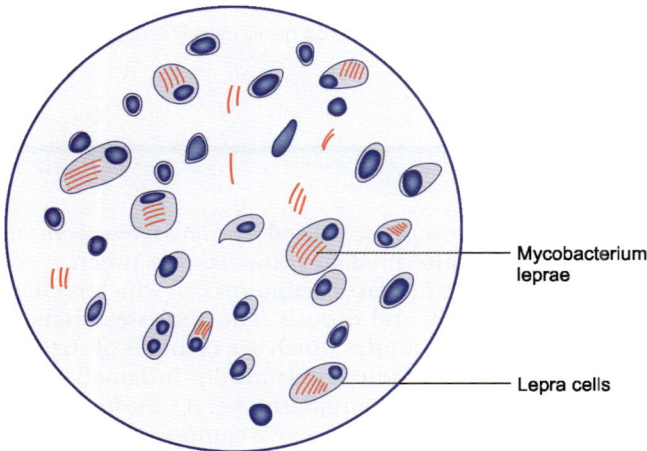

Figure 16.5 *Mycobacterium leprae* — straight or slightly curved acid-fast bacilli (bright red in colour).

either intracellularly or lying free outside the cell. These are present as bundles or clumps of bacilli in a lipid-like capsular material known as glia. These masses, known as globi and the bacilli arranged in parallel rows within the globi, have a cigar-bundle appearance. The *globi (masses of bacilli)*, which are *seen within the histiocytes*, have a foamy appearance and are *known as lepra cells.*

CORYNEBACTERIUM DIPHTHERIAE

C. diphtheriae is a thin, *slender*, non–acid-fast, *Gram-positive bacillus* that *causes diphtheria.* The bacilli are pleomorphic. These bacilli have a tendency to clubbing at one or both ends. The *bacilli are usually arranged in angular fashion resembling letters V or L* (Fig. 16.6). They *are* club-shaped due to the *presence of metachromatic granules at one or both ends.* These granules are known as *Babes-Ernst bodies.* The *bacilli* are *stained* green and metachromatic granules bluish-black with *Albert stain.*

Metachromasia: The property of certain biological materials of staining a different colour from that of the stain used.

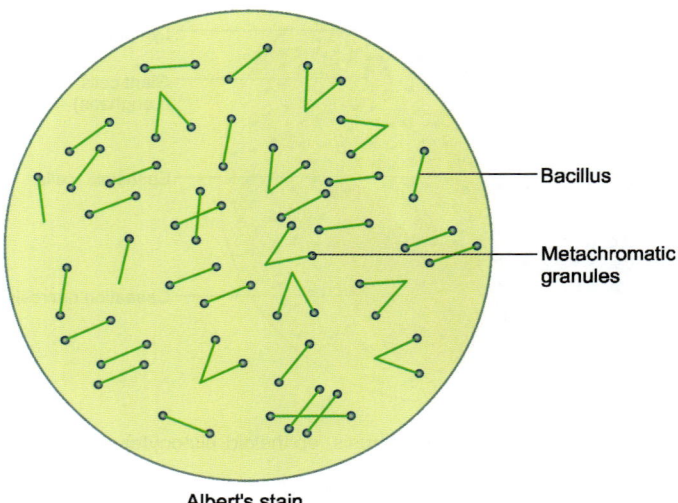

Albert's stain

Figure 16.6 *Corynebacterium diphtheriae* — green coloured bacilli usually arranged in letters V or L with bluish-black metachromatic granules at the ends.

ACTINOMYCOSIS

Actinomycosis is a chronic granulomatous infection caused by *filamentous, branching Gram-positive bacteria* known as 'actinomycetes' (having intermediate properties between true bacteria and fungi) (Fig. 16.7). In humans, *Actinomyces israelii* causes actinomycosis which is characterized by multiple abscesses and sinuses, tissue destruction and fibrosis. The abscesses discharging pus usually contain yellowish flecks known as sulphur granules which are colonies of *Actinomyces*. In tissues, there is a peripheral band of fibrosis surrounding chronically inflamed granulation tissue, large number of neutrophils and colonies of microorganism, i.e. *A. israelii*. In the H&E-stained section, the *individual colony* appear as *rounded or lobulated masses* composed of *meshwork of filaments* (central core) *that stain basophilic* and *club-shaped ends (peripherally)* of filaments that *stain eosinophilic.*

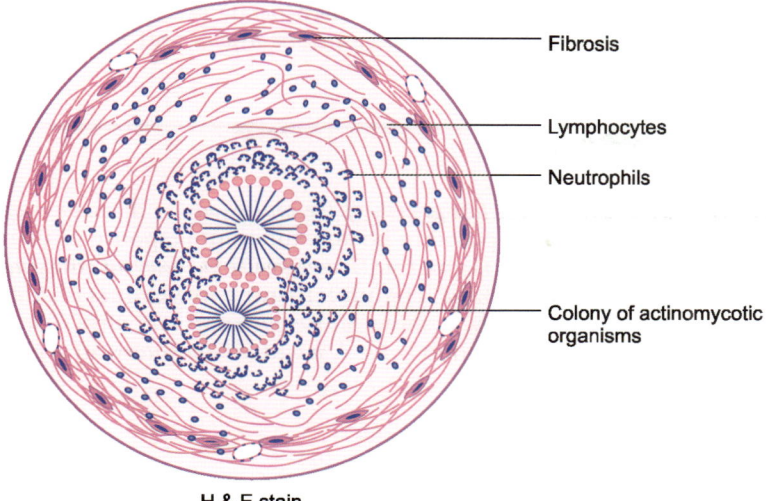

H & E stain

Figure 16.7 Actinomycosis — peripheral fibrosis, lymphocytes and large number of neutrophils with colony of acti-nomycotic organisms. The individual colony appears as rounded mass of basophilic filaments and eosinophilic club-shaped ends.

This particular appearance of colony with characteristic peripheral radiating filaments is often called as '*ray fungus*'. Multinucleated giant cells and macrophages are often seen around the periphery of the lesion.

CANDIDA ALBICANS

C. albicans is a yeast-like *fungus* causing an *opportunistic endogenous infection, candidosis* (Fig. 16.8). It is a component of normal, oral and body flora. It is a *Gram-positive ovoid or spherical budding cell*

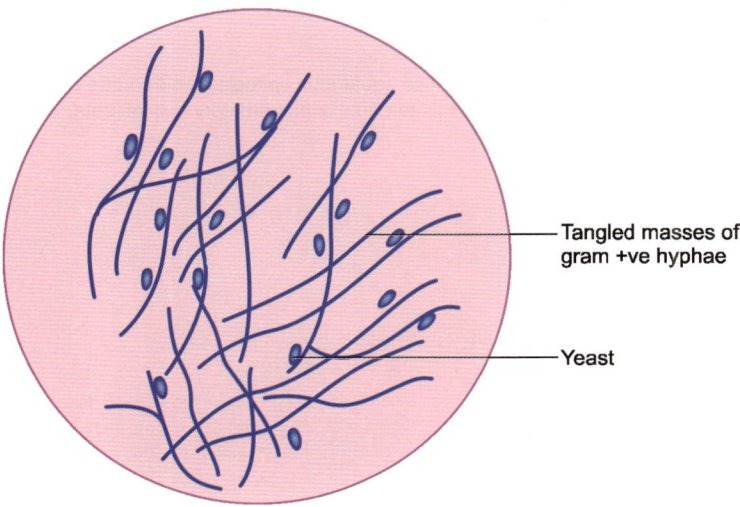

Figure 16.8 *Candida albicans* — tangled masses of Gram-positive hyphae and yeast.

which produces pseudomycelia. *Unicellular fungi* which occur *as spherical or ovoid cells are yeasts. Tubular or thread-like structures formed by elongation of cell are hyphae* and *tangled masses of hyphae* are known as *mycelium.*

PYOGENIC GRANULOMA

Pyogenic granuloma is a *common tumour-like growth of the oral cavity* as a *response of the tissues to the nonspecific infection* (Fig. 16.9). It is supposed to be an exuberant response of tissue to local irritation or trauma. The most common site is gingiva. *Histologically, it shows an overlying epithelium which may be thin or hyperplastic or may be ulcerated.* The underlying *connective tissue stroma is delicate with proliferation of fibroblast.* Characteristically, it shows *numerous small and large endothelium-lined blood capillaries* which are engorged with red blood cells. A *mixed inflammatory cell infiltrate of neutrophils, plasma cells and lymphocytes* is seen.

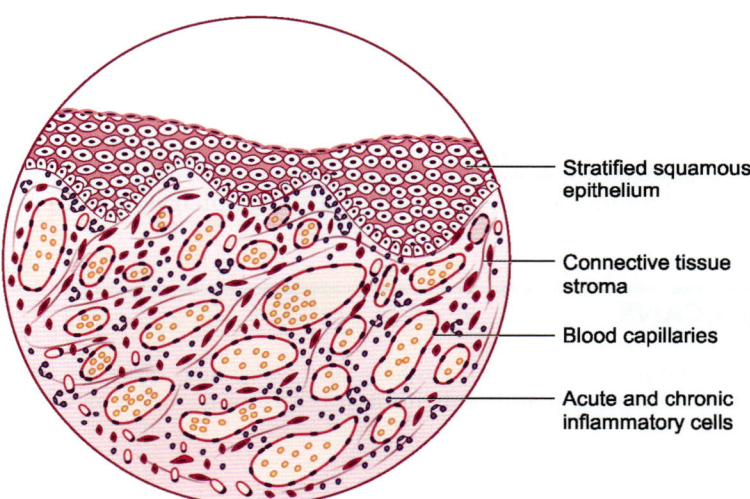

Stratified squamous epithelium

Connective tissue stroma

Blood capillaries

Acute and chronic inflammatory cells

Figure 16.9 Pyogenic granuloma — overlying stratified squamous epithelium, numerous small and large endothelium-lined blood capillaries engorged with RBCs and a mixed chronic inflammatory cell infiltrate.

Dental Caries | 17

PIT AND FISSURE CARIES

Pit and fissure caries is a primary *type of dental caries* according to morphology or anatomical site of the lesion on an individual tooth (Fig. 17.1). It affects the occlusal surface of *premolars and molars*, buccal and lingual surface of molars and palatal surface of maxillary incisors. It *appears as a triangular or cone-shaped lesion* with the *base towards the dentinoenamel junction* and the *apex at the outer surface.* It generally follows the direction of enamel rods. There is undermining of enamel through the lateral spread of caries at the dentinoenamel junction. In longitudinal

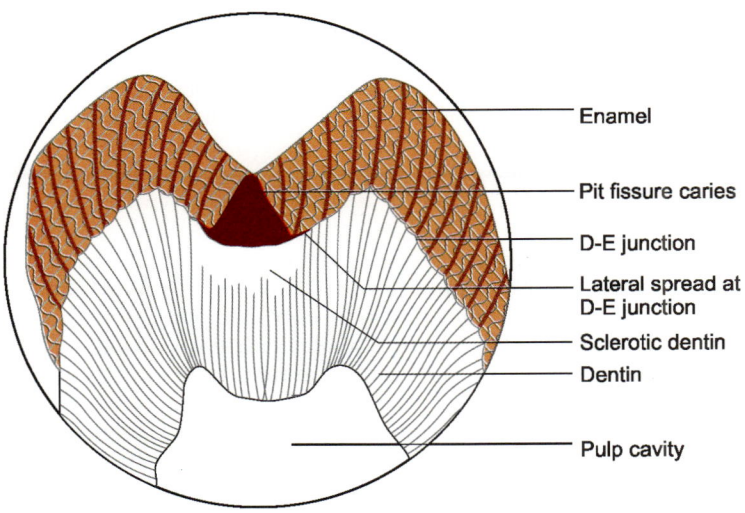

Enamel

Pit fissure caries

D-E junction

Lateral spread at D-E junction

Sclerotic dentin

Dentin

Pulp cavity

Figure 17.1 Pit and fissure caries (GS) — appears as a triangular or cone-shaped lesion with the base towards the dentinoenamel junction and the apex at the outer surface.

ground section under light microscope, initial carious lesion shows four different zones starting from the inner advancing front of the lesion: (i) translucent zone, (ii) dark zone, (iii) body of lesion and (iv) surface zone.

SMOOTH SURFACE CARIES

Smooth surface caries is the primary type of *dental caries* according to the morphology or anatomical site of lesion on an individual tooth (Fig. 17.2). It affects the proximal surfaces of the *teeth or the gingival third of the* buccal or lingual surfaces. In early lesions (i) there is loss of interprismatic or inter-rod substance with increased prominence of rods; (ii) there is accentuation of incremental lines of Retzius (optical phenomenon due to loss of minerals so that there is more prominence of organic structures); and (iii) there may be accentuation of perikymata which are external manifestation of striae of Retzius. It *appears as a triangular or cone-shaped lesion with the base near the surface of tooth and the apex towards the dentinoenamel junction.*

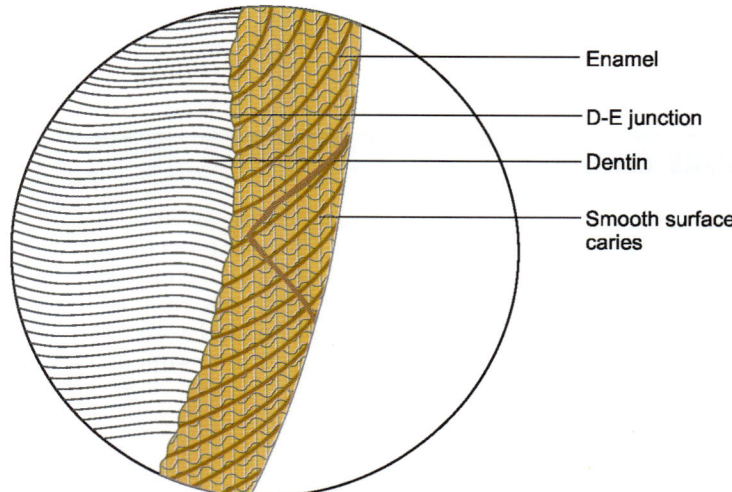

Enamel

D-E junction

Dentin

Smooth surface caries

Figure 17.2 Smooth surface caries (GS) — appears as a cone-shaped lesion on the proximal surface of the tooth with the base near the surface of the tooth and the apex towards the dentinoenamel junction.

CARIES IN DENTIN

Caries in dentin starts as there is a natural process of spread of dental caries along the dentinoenamel junction and the rapid involvement of dentinal tubules (Fig. 17.3). Early dentinal changes are dentinal sclerosis and fatty degeneration of odontoblastic processes. Fatty degeneration may favour the sclerosis of dentinal tubules. There is a decalcification of wall of the dentinal tubules and migration of microorganisms within the tubules, so that these tubules get distended and have the beaded appearance.

Advanced dentinal changes show the confluence of individual dentinal tubules due to the decalcification of walls of the dentinal tubules. There is a *focal coalescence and breakdown of few dentinal tubules* which form a *tiny liquefaction foci as described by Miller.* It appears as an *ovoid area of destruction* filled with *necrotic debris* and runs parallel to the direction of the tubules. The *extension of carious process* along the *lateral branches of the dentinal tubules* and *along the matrix fibres leads* to the *formation of clefts* which are at right angle *to the dentinal tubules.*

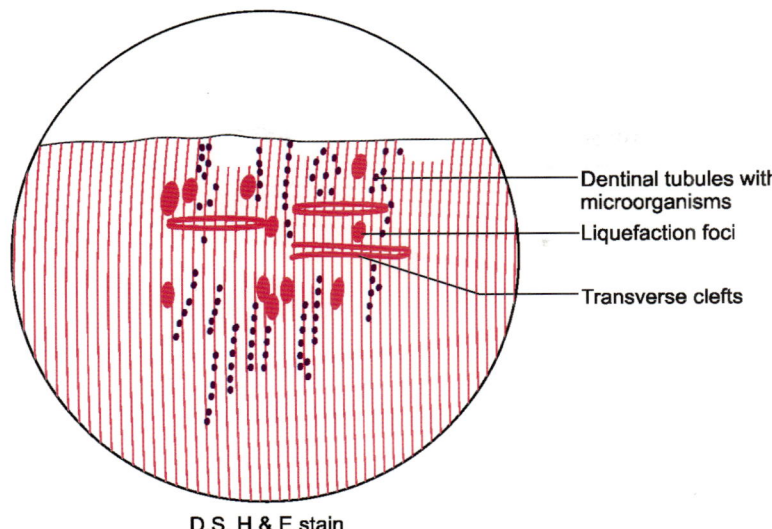

Dentinal tubules with microorganisms

Liquefaction foci

Transverse clefts

D.S. H & E stain

Figure 17.3 Caries in dentin — dentinal tubules containing microorganisms, transverse clefts and liquefaction foci of Miller.

As there is a progression of the carious lesion, various zones in the carious dentin beginning pulpally are as follows:

Zone 1 – zone of fatty degeneration of odontoblastic processes
Zone 2 – zone of dentinal sclerosis
Zone 3 – zone of decalcification of dentin
Zone 4 – zone of bacterial invasion of decalcified but intact dentin
Zone 5 – zone of decomposed dentin

Chapter 12

Figure 12.1 ...

Zone 1 —
Zone 2 —
Zone 3 —
Zone 4 —

Diseases of Pulp and Periapical Tissues

18

ACUTE PULPITIS

Acute pulpitis is an *inflammation of the pulp* due to injury to the pulp, usually from dental caries or trauma (Fig. 18.1). *Histologically,* it shows the *dilatation of blood vessels* and accumulation of oedema fluid. In early lesion, there is *localized infiltration* of acute *inflammatory cells,* mostly the *polymorphonuclear leukocytes.* Localized destruction leads to the formation of a small abscess known as *pulp abscess,* which is a circumscribed area containing pus resulting from the break-down of leukocytes, bacteria and digestion of tissue. As inflammation spreads, most of the pulp is infiltrated by the polymorphonuclear leukocytes. There is a *degeneration of the odontoblastic layer.*

CHRONIC PULPITIS

Chronic pulpitis may be the *sequelae of a previous acute pulpitis* or occurs *as a chronic type of disease from the onset* (Fig. 18.2). *Histologically,* there is a *diffuse infiltration of pulp tissue by mononuclear cells,* chiefly lymphocytes and plasma cells in a variable number. Blood capillaries are numerous. *Collagen fibres are seen in bundles* with prominent fibroblastic activity. The tissue reaction results in the formation of granulation tissue. *There is a loss of odontoblastic layer.*

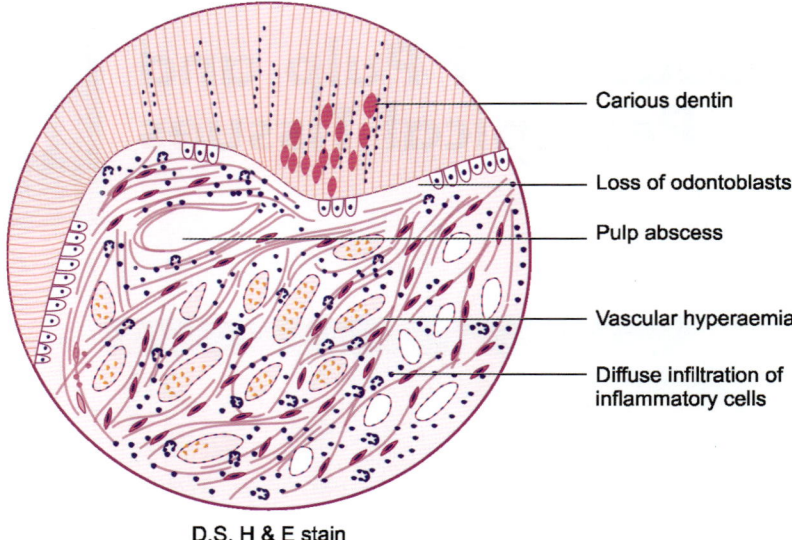

Carious dentin

Loss of odontoblasts

Pulp abscess

Vascular hyperaemia

Diffuse infiltration of inflammatory cells

D.S. H & E stain

Figure 18.1 Acute pulpitis — carious lesion in the dentin and pulp with diffused infiltration by polymorphonuclear leukocytes, formation of pulp abscess and degeneration of odontoblastic layer.

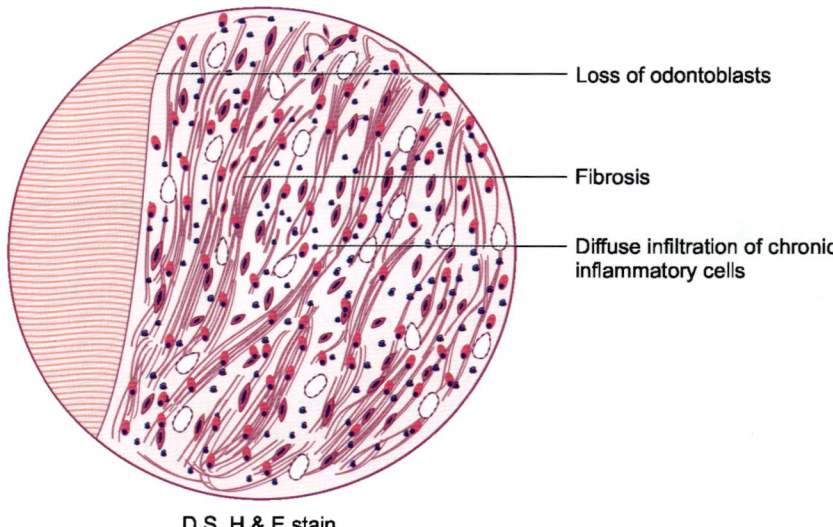

Loss of odontoblasts

Fibrosis

Diffuse infiltration of chronic inflammatory cells

D.S. H & E stain

Figure 18.2 Chronic pulpitis – diffuse infiltration of pulp by chronic inflammatory cells – lymphocytes and plasma cells, fibrosis and loss of odontoblastic layer.

CHRONIC HYPERPLASTIC PULPITIS (PULP POLYP)

Chronic hyperplastic pulpitis is a *unique type of chronic pulpitis* that *occurs in children and young adults* with *high pulp tissue resistance and reactivity* (Fig. 18.3). It is *characterized by formation of granulation tissue covered by stratified squamous epithelium.* This granulation tissue consists of delicate collagen fibres, proliferation of fibroblasts and variable number of small blood capillaries. The inflammatory cell infiltration consists chiefly of lymphocytes and plasma cells with few polymorphonuclear

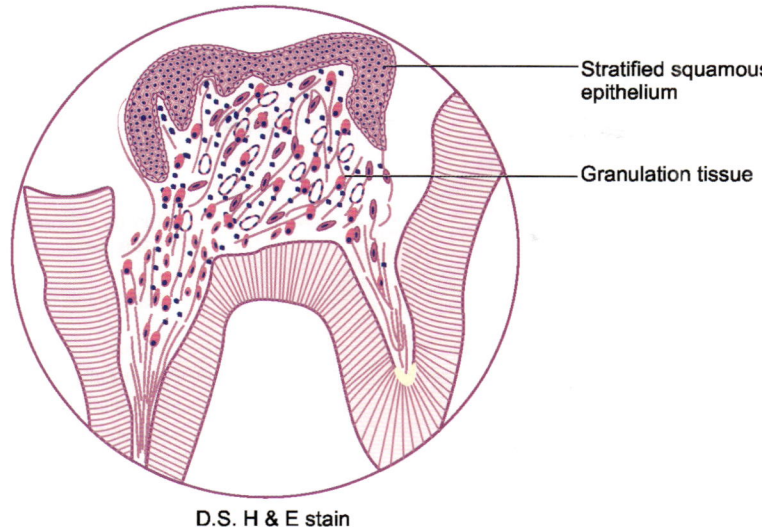

D.S. H & E stain

Figure 18.3   Chronic hyperplastic pulpitis — granulation tissue covered by stratified squamous epithelium.

leukocytes. This *granulation tissue* is *covered with stratified squamous epithelium* as a result of implantation of epithelial cells from oral mucous membrane.

PULP NECROSIS

Complete necrosis of pulp tissue is the *sequelae of untreated acute or chronic pulpitis* (Fig. 18.4). It can also be known as pulp gangrene as the *necrosis of pulp* is generally *associated with bacterial infection.*

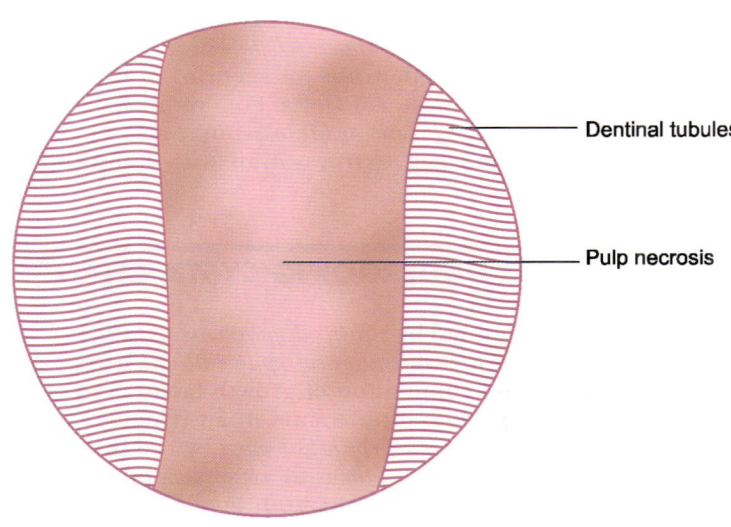

D.S. H & E stain

Figure 18.4   Pulp necrosis – necrosis of pulp.

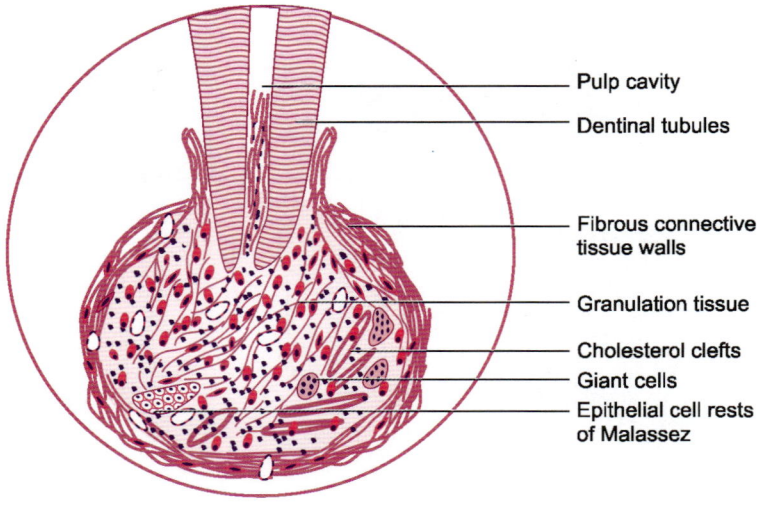

Pulp cavity

Dentinal tubules

Fibrous connective
tissue walls

Granulation tissue

Cholesterol clefts

Giant cells

Epithelial cell rests
of Malassez

D.S. H & E stain

Figure 18.5 Periapical granuloma – periapical granuloma surrounded by connective tissue capsule and shows delicate fibrillar stroma, fibroblastic proliferation, dense chronic inflammatory cell infiltrate, cholesterol clefts with giant cells and epithelial cell rests of Malassez.

PERIAPICAL GRANULOMA (CHRONIC APICAL PERIODONTITIS)

Periapical granuloma is a *localized mass of chronic granulation tissue* at the *apex of root* of a *non-vital tooth* as a response to infection (Fig. 18.5). *Histologically,* it shows a *granulation tissue surrounded by fibrous connective tissue capsule.* Granulation tissue consists of delicate fibrillar stroma with fibroblastic proliferation and variably dense lymphocytic and plasma cell infiltration intermixed frequently with neutrophils and histiocytes and less frequently with mast cells and eosinophils. There is a presence of numerous small blood capillaries. *Cholesterol crystal/clefts* represented as *clear needle-like spaces/clefts* which are due to dissolution of cholesterol by the agents used during preparation of section. *Multinucleated foreign body giant cells* may be associated with these cholesterol clefts. Foci of lipid–laden macrophages (foam cell) are sometimes seen. *Epithelial cell rests of Malassez* may also be seen within the periapical granuloma. Areas of red blood cell extravasation with hemosiderin pigment may be present.

PERIAPICAL GRANULOMA UNDERGOING CYSTIC CHANGE

It is *a process* by which a *cystic cavity* lined by *stratified squamous epithelium* with a connective tissue wall *develops* (Fig. 18.6). There is a *proliferation of epithelial cell rests of Malassez* incorporated within the granuloma as a result of stimulation of growth factors released by a variety of cells present in the granuloma. This proliferation occurs in an irregular pattern. *Due to continued epithelial proliferation,* there is *an increase in epithelial mass* by the division of basal cells on the periphery. Thus, the *cells in the central part of the mass are* separated *away from their source of nutrition.* As these *central cells do not get* sufficient nutrition, they *degenerate* and become *necrotic and liquefy.* This *forms an epithelial* lined *cystic cavity* filled with fluid.

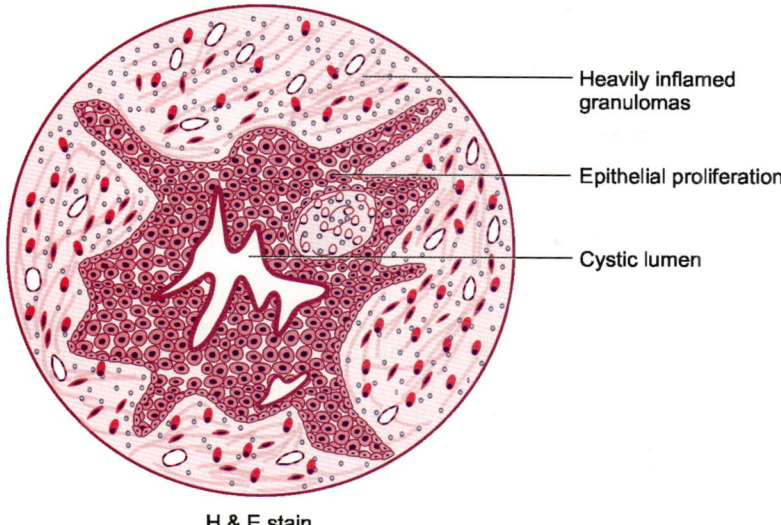

H & E stain

Figure 18.6 Periapical granuloma undergoing cystic change — a cystic lumen in the centre and adjacent granuloma.

RADICULAR CYST (APICAL PERIODONTAL CYST, PERIAPICAL CYST)

Radicular cyst is the most *common epithelial* lined *odontogenic cyst of inflammatory origin* (Fig. 18.7). *Histologically*, it shows *a cystic lumen* lined *by stratified squamous epithelium of variable thickness.* This epithelial lining may be discontinuous or missing over the areas of intense inflammation. *Occasionally* this *lining epithelium* may show the *presence of tiny linear* or

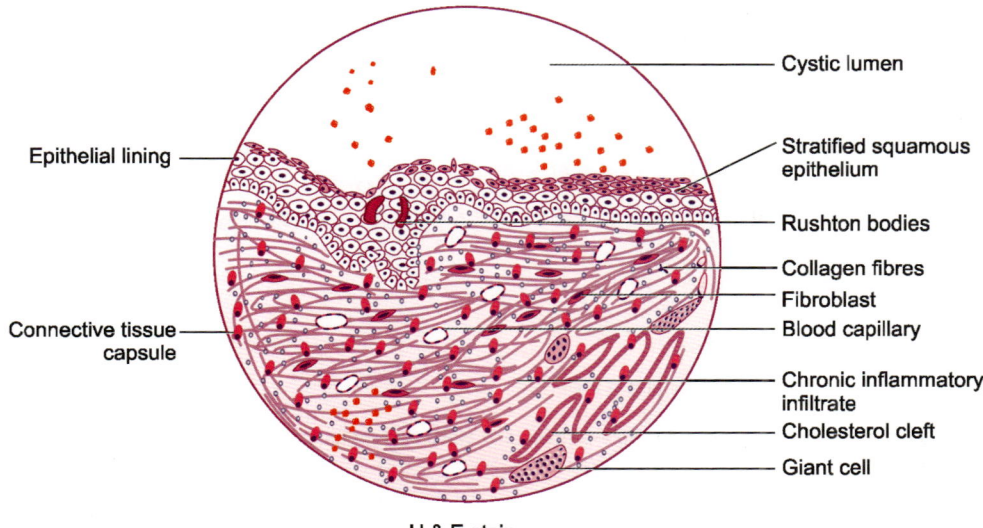

H & E stain

Figure 18.7 Radicular cyst — cystic lumen by stratified squamous epithelium with arc-shaped eosinophilic Rushton bodies and underlying connective tissue capsule with dense chronic inflammatory cell infiltrate, cholesterol clefts and giant cells.

arc-shaped bodies known as *Rushton bodies* which are amorphous in structure, eosinophilic in reaction and brittle in nature. The *underlying fibrous connective tissue capsule* is composed of *condensed parallel bundles of collagen fibres* with variable number of fibroblasts and small blood capillaries. *Presence of inflammatory cell infiltrate* in the connective tissue immediately adjacent to the overlying epithelium *is a characteristic feature.* This inflammatory cell infiltrate is composed of lymphocytes and plasma cells with admixture of polymorphonuclear leukocytes and foamy macrophages. Dystrophic calcifications, *cholesterol clefts associated* with *multinucleated giant cells,* red blood cells and areas of haemorrhage may be seen in the cystic wall or lumen or both. The cystic lumen contains watery, straw-coloured, blood-tinged fluid and cellular debris.

CHOLESTEROL CLEFTS AND GIANT CELLS

Histologically cholesterol clefts are seen in many but not all periapical granulomas or radicular cysts (Fig. 18.8). They *appear as clear needle-like spaces or clefts* due to dissolution of cholesterol within them during the processing of tissue for microscopic examination. The source of this cholesterol is not known, although it has been suggested that the local tissue damage is essential for cholesterol deposition. These are often seen in areas with inflammation and may be derived from inflammatory cells, or breakdown of extravasated red blood cells. These cholesterol clefts are almost associated with foreign body type of multinucleated giant cells.

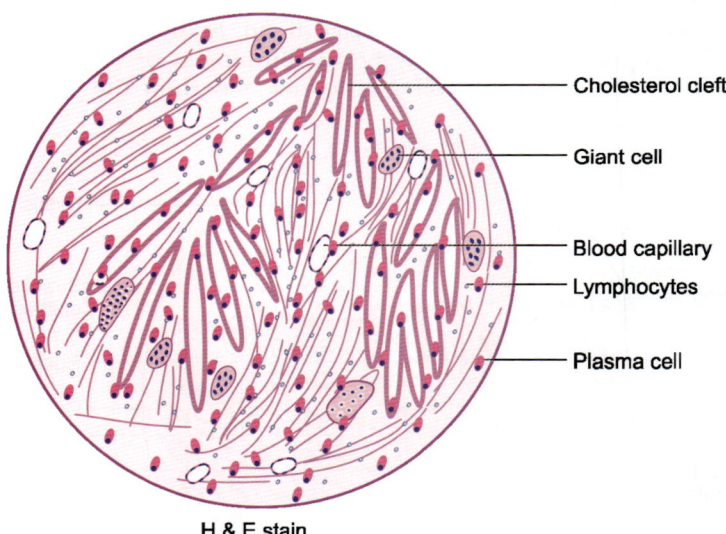

Cholesterol cleft

Giant cell

Blood capillary
Lymphocytes

Plasma cell

H & E stain

Figure 18.8   Cholesterol clefts and giant cells — cholesterol clefts appear as clear needle-like spaces and multinucleated giant cells.

SEQUESTRUM

A *sequestrum is a fragment of the necrotic* (dead) *bone* which is separated from the adjacent vital bone (Fig. 18.9). In acute suppurative osteomyelitis, there is an acute inflammation of marrow tissue and subsequent spread of inflammatory exudate through the marrow spaces. This is followed by vascular compression, thrombosis and obstruction of blood flow, and ultimately necrosis of bone. *Histologically, this necrotic bone* shows *loss of osteocytes* from the *lacunae*. These sequestra may get exfoliated spontaneously. Occasionally, these fragments of necrotic bone may be surrounded by a new vital bone known as involucrum.

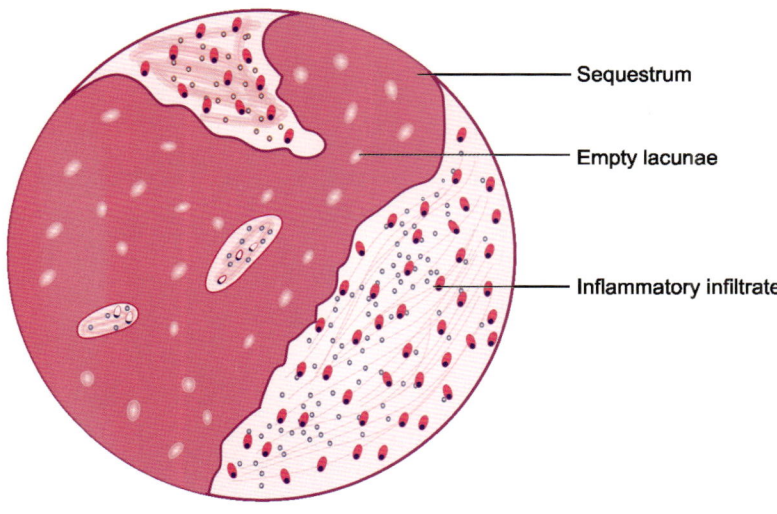

Sequestrum

Empty lacunae

Inflammatory infiltrate

D.S. H & E stain

Figure 18.9   Sequestrum — necrotic bone with loss of osteocytes from the lacunae and inflammation of marrow tissue.

Diseases of Bones **19**

FIBROUS DYSPLASIA

Fibrous dysplasia is *nonhereditary, developmental tumour-like condition of the bone characterized* by *replacement of the normal bone* by a *cellular fibrous connective tissue* with *formation of secondary metaplastic bone* (Fig. 19.1). Mono-ostotic fibrous dysplasia of jaw bones typically *consists* of *loose cellular fibrous stroma* with *irregular, slender and discrete C-shaped or Chinese letter pattern* of *trabeculae of immature (woven) bone*. These bony trabeculae are supposed to be formed by metaplasia and do not show osteoblastic rimming. The *fibrous connective tissue* is *mild to moderately cellular* with mononuclear cells resembling fibroblasts and progenitor osteoblasts. The lesional tissue merges directly with

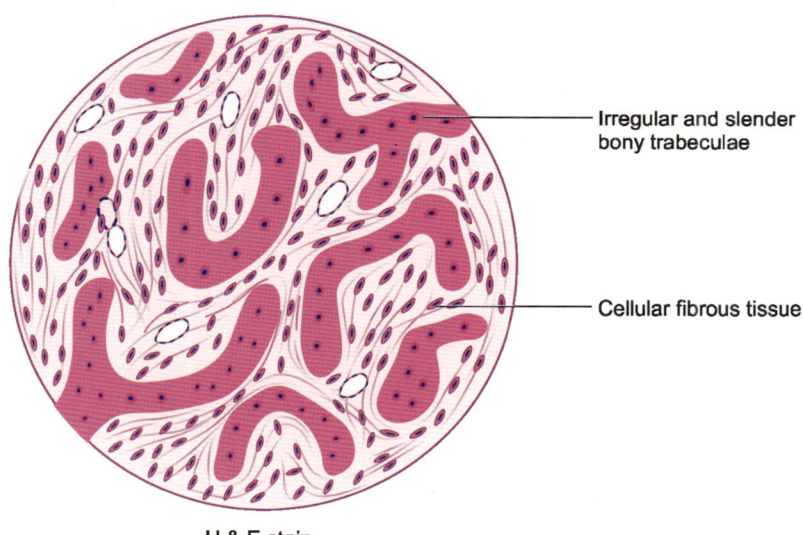

Irregular and slender bony trabeculae

Cellular fibrous tissue

H & E stain

Figure 19.1 Fibrous dysplasia — irregularly shaped bony trabeculae of woven bone in a loose, cellular fibrous connective tissue stroma. These trabeculae are without osteoblastic rimming.

the adjacent normal bone, so the capsule is absent. As the lesion matures, it shows the presence of lamellar bone in a moderate cellular connective tissue stroma.

PAGET DISEASE (OSTEITIS DEFORMANS)

Paget disease is a chronic *progressive disorder characterized* by *abnormal and disorganized resorption and deposition of bone* (Fig. 19.2). *Histologically,* it *shows rapid resorption and new bone formation.* During resorption, bony trabeculae are surrounded by numerous osteoclasts (abnormally large cells with many nuclei). Simultaneously, osteoblastic activity is evident, resulting in formation of bony trabeculae with osteoid rims. A *characteristic feature is the presence of basophilic reversal lines* in the bone, indicative of the junction between alternative/repeated bone resorption and bone formation. This gives a '*jigsaw puzzle*' or *mosaic appearance* to the bone. The marrow is replaced by highly vascular fibrous connective tissue.

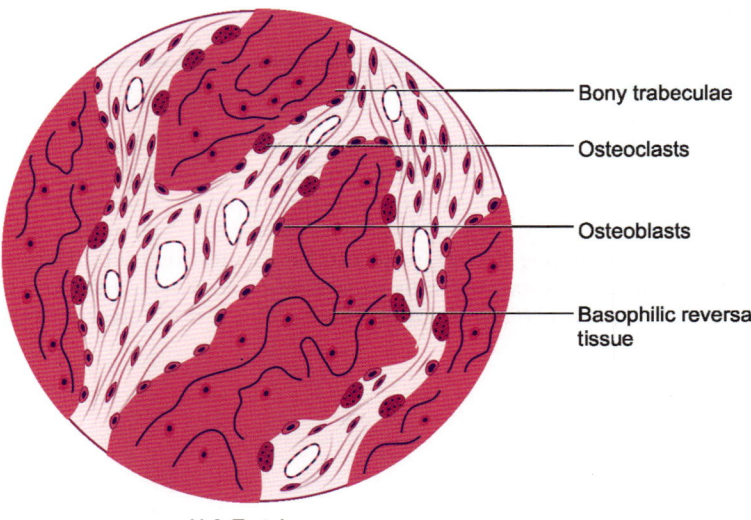

Bony trabeculae

Osteoclasts

Osteoblasts

Basophilic reversal tissue

H & E stain

Figure 19.2 Paget disease — bony trabeculae with prominent osteoblastic and osteoclastic activity and resting and reversal lines.

Diseases of Skin 20

ORAL LICHEN PLANUS

Lichen planus is a *relatively common chronic autoimmune mucocutaneous disease* that frequently affects the oral mucosa (Fig. 20.1). The histopathological features are typical but not always specific. The *stratified squamous epithelium* shows *varying degrees of hyperorthokeratosis* or *hyperparakeratosis* depending on the form of lichen planus. The *spinous cell layer may* be of *variable thickness.* The *rete ridges* have a *'saw tooth'* or *pointed appearance* which is more common in nonoral forms of lichen planus. *Degeneration of the basal cell layer of* the *epithelium* is seen. *Degenerating basal cells* form *colloid, civatte, hyaline or cytoid bodies* which are seen as homogeneous eosinophilic globules at epithelium and connective

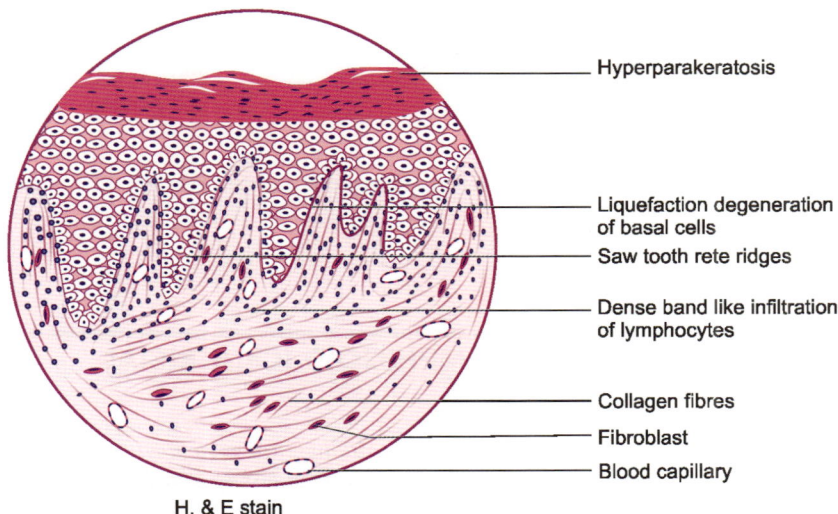

Hyperparakeratosis

Liquefaction degeneration of basal cells

Saw tooth rete ridges

Dense band like infiltration of lymphocytes

Collagen fibres

Fibroblast

Blood capillary

H. & E stain

Figure 20.1   Oral lichen planus — hyperparakeratosis, saw tooth rete ridges, liquefaction degeneration of basal cell layer and dense band-like infiltration of lymphocytes.

123

tissue interface. There is a dense band-like chronic inflammatory cell infiltrate predominantly of lymphocytes (T-lymphocytes) in the superficial lamina propria immediately subadjacent to the epithelium.

PEMPHIGUS VULGARIS

Pemphigus vulgaris is a *chronic, autoimmune vesiculobullous disease* affecting skin and mucous membranes (Fig. 20.2). *Microscopically*, it is *characterized* by *intraepithelial vesicle* or *bulla formation just above the basal cell layer* with *suprabasilar split*. The cells of the spinous cell layer lose their attachment which is called *acantholysis* or *loss of cohesiveness*. These loose cells become rounded in shape and the cytoplasm around the nucleus contracts with swelling of the nuclei and hyperchromatic staining. These cells are known as *Tzanck cells* and are found in small groups within a vesicle. The underlying connective tissue is fibrocellular with mild to moderate chronic inflammatory cell infiltrate.

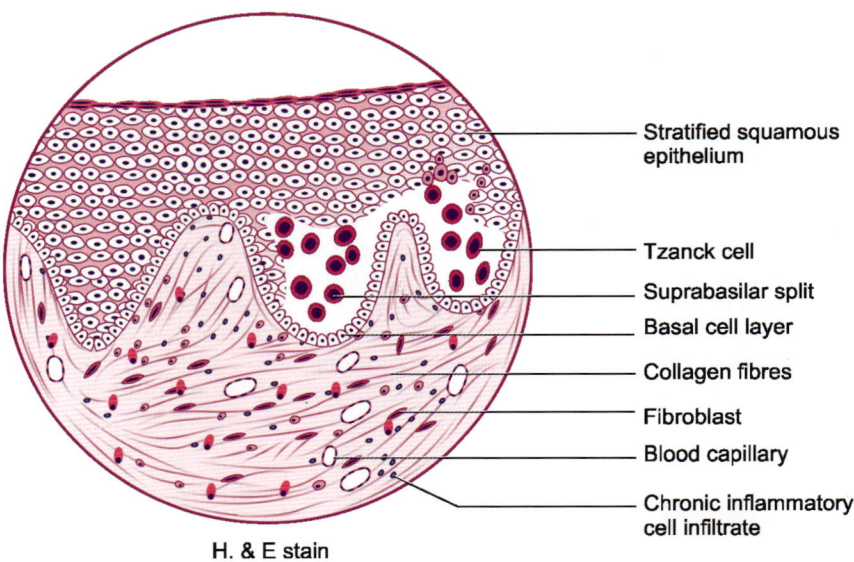

Stratified squamous epithelium

Tzanck cell

Suprabasilar split

Basal cell layer

Collagen fibres

Fibroblast

Blood capillary

Chronic inflammatory cell infiltrate

H. & E stain

Figure 20.2 Pemphigus vulgaris — intraepithelial cleft just above the basal cell layer with Tzanck cells which appear as rounded cells with hyperchromatic staining.

BENIGN MUCOUS MEMBRANE PEMPHIGOID (CICATRICIAL PEMPHIGOID)

Benign mucous membrane pemphigoid is an *uncommon autoimmune vesiculobullous disease* (Fig. 20.3). The *vesicles and bullae are subepithelial histologically*. There is *loss of attachment of surface epithelium* and the *underlying connective tissue* and thus *separation of full thickness of epithelium* from the connective *tissue at the basement membrane level*. There is no acantholysis. The roof of the bulla is formed by the epithelium and the floor by the connective tissue which is infiltrated by nonspecific chronic inflammatory infiltrate of lymphocytes, plasma cells and eosinophils.

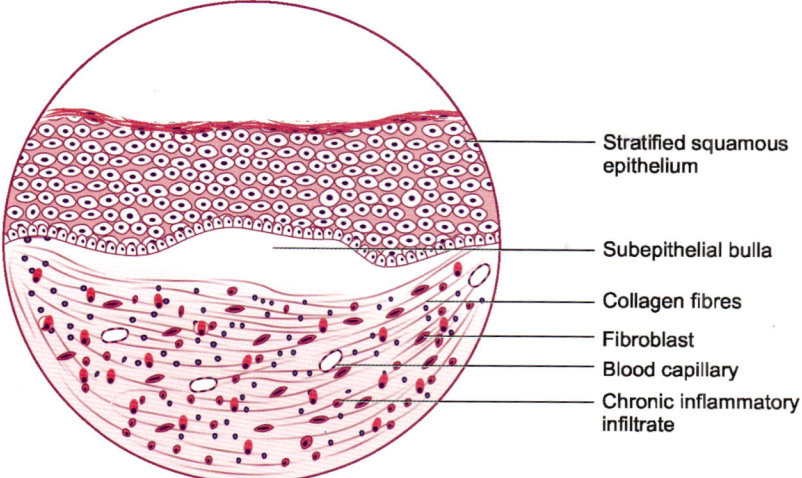

Figure 20.3 Benign mucous membrane pemphigoid — subepithelial cleft resulting in separation of the epithelium from the underlying connective tissue.

ERYTHEMA MULTIFORME

Erythema multiforme is an *acute blistering, ulcerative* and *self-limiting mucocutaneous condition* of uncertain aetiology, possibly mediated immunologically (Fig. 20.4). The histological features are variable. Vesicles or bullae are subepithelial or intraepithelial. There is a necrosis of the basal keratinocytes. The *underlying connective tissue* shows *varying degrees of mixed inflammatory cell infiltration*, chiefly of lymphocytes but also of neutrophils and eosinophils and may have a *perivascular distribution*. There may be dilatation of superficial blood capillaries and lymphatic vessels in upper part of the connective tissue.

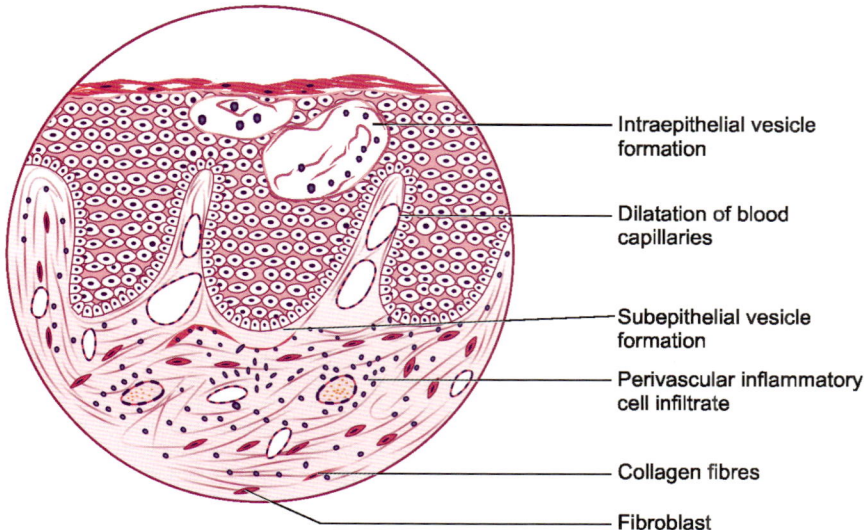

Figure 20.4 Erythema multiforme — intraepithelial and subepithelial vesicle formation with perivascular inflammatory cell infiltrate.

Cysts of Nonodontogenic Origin

21

NASOPALATINE DUCT CYST (INCISIVE CANAL CYST)

Nasopalatine duct cyst is the *nonodontogenic developmental cyst* which often occurs in the midline of palate in anterior maxilla (Fig. 21.1). *Histologically,* it shows a *cystic lumen lined by epithelium* which may be *stratified squamous, pseudostratified columnar, simple columnar or cuboidal type.* These may be there within the same cyst. The *fibrous cyst wall* characteristically *shows the presence of blood vessels* and *nerves* which are from neurovascular bundles normally passing through incisive canal. Small mucous glands and adipose tissue may also be seen. Mild to dense chronic inflammatory cell

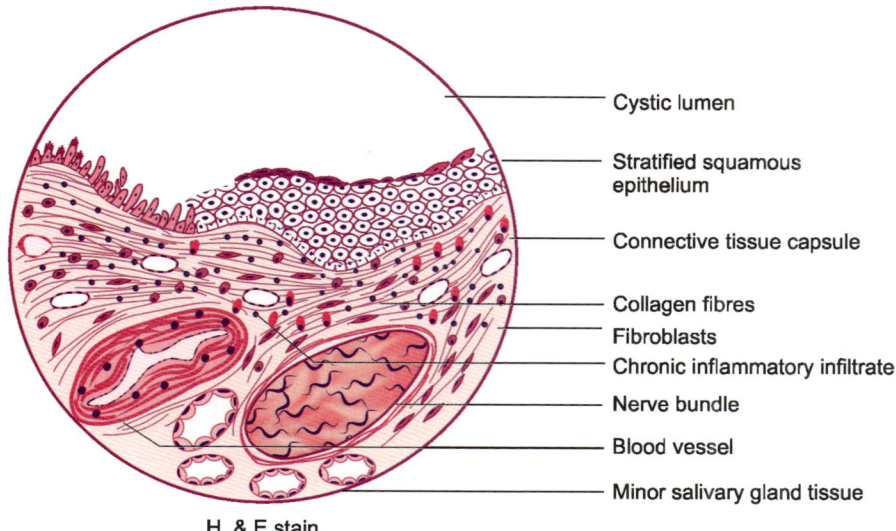

Cystic lumen

Stratified squamous epithelium

Connective tissue capsule

Collagen fibres
Fibroblasts
Chronic inflammatory infiltrate
Nerve bundle
Blood vessel
Minor salivary gland tissue

H. & E stain

Figure 21.1 Nasopalatine duct cyst — cystic lumen lined by stratified squamous epithelium and the cyst wall with the presence of blood vessel, nerve bundle and minor salivary gland tissue.

infiltration of lymphocytes and plasma cells is often seen. The cyst fluid is straw coloured and composed of leukocytes, erythrocytes, desquamated epithelial cells, tissue debris and microorganisms.

THYROGLOSSAL DUCT CYST (THYROGLOSSAL TRACT CYST)

Thyroglossal duct cyst is a rare *nonodontogenic developmental cyst* which *occurs usually in the midline of neck* but may occur anywhere from foramen caecum of the tongue to the suprasternal notch (Fig. 21.2). *Histologically, it shows a cystic cavity lined by stratified squamous, ciliated columnar or intermediate transition type of epithelium.* The underlying connective tissue wall shows the *presence of thyroid tissue,* small patches of lymphoid tissue and mucous glands.

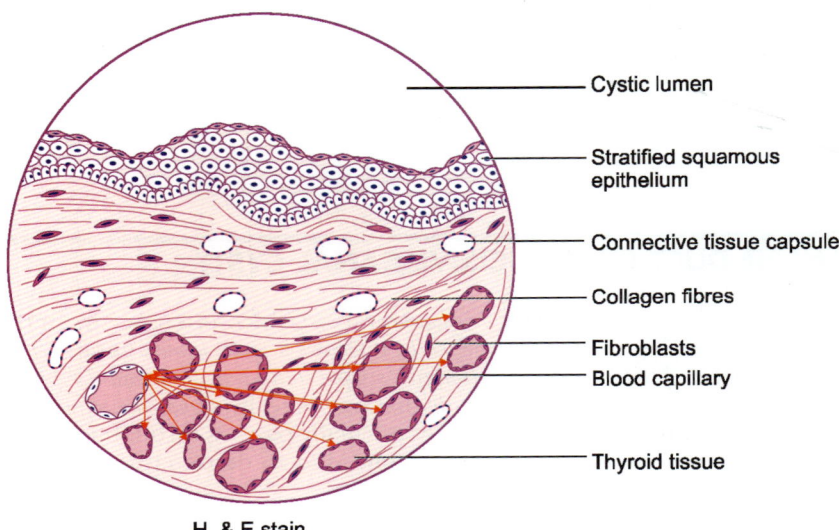

H. & E stain

Figure 21.2   Thyroglossal duct cyst — cystic lumen lined by stratified squamous epithelium with thyroid follicles in the connective tissue wall.

MUCOCELE

Mucocele is a *nonodontogenic* cyst of *salivary gland origin* (Fig. 21.3). It usually results from rupture of salivary gland duct and obstruction to the drainage of minor salivary gland. Two distinct entities of mucocele have been described.

Mucous Extravasation Type

This is *most commonly seen* on the *lower lip* due to the rupture of minor salivary gland duct produced by the biting of lips and there is spillage of mucin into the surrounding soft tissue (Fig. 21.3A). *Histologically, it consists of circumscribed cavity* in *submucosal connective tissue* causing an obvious elevation of the overlying mucosa with thinning of the epithelium. As the cystic cavity is not lined by the epithelium, it is *not a true cyst.* The *wall is* made up of *lining of compressed fibrous connective tissue and fibroblasts.* Usually this connective tissue wall is actually granulation tissue, thus with infiltration of abundant polymorphonuclear lymphocytes, lymphocytes and plasma cells. The cystic lumen is filled with eosinophilic coagulum with variable number of leukocytes and

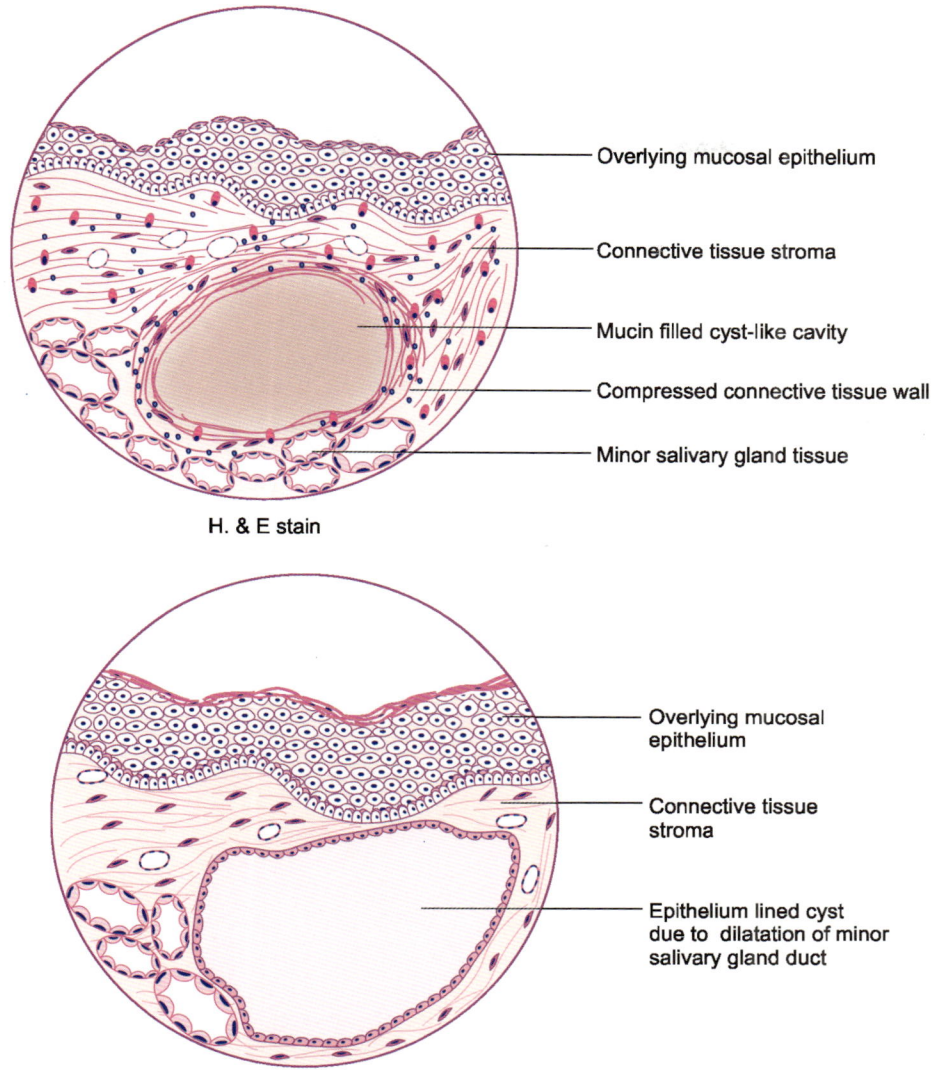

H. & E stain

- Overlying mucosal epithelium
- Connective tissue stroma
- Mucin filled cyst-like cavity
- Compressed connective tissue wall
- Minor salivary gland tissue

H. & E stain

- Overlying mucosal epithelium
- Connective tissue stroma
- Epithelium lined cyst due to dilatation of minor salivary gland duct

Figure 21.3 (A) Mucocele – mucous extravasation cyst – mucin-filled cyst cavity lined by compressed fibrous connective tissue with granulation tissue and adjacent minor salivary gland tissue. (B) Mucocele – mucous retention cyst – cystic cavity lined by cuboidal epithelium due to gross dilation of minor salivary gland duct and overlying mucosal epithelium.

mononuclear phagocytes. The *adjacent minor salivary gland tissue* often shows a *chronic inflammatory cell infiltrate* and *dilated ducts*.

Mucous Retention Type

It is an *epithelium-lined cavity* which arises from *salivary gland tissue* due to the obstruction of salivary gland duct so that the duct becomes distended (Fig. 21.3B). The *lining of* this dilated *duct is variable – cuboidal, columnar or atrophic squamous epithelium*. Salivary *gland tissue* may *be seen*.

Bibliography

1. **Orban's**
   GS Kumar, SN Bhaskar. Orban's Oral Histology and Embryology. 14th ed. New Delhi: Elsevier; 2015.
2. **Ten Cate's**
   A Nanci. Ten Cate's Oral Histology – Development, Structure and Function. 8th ed. St Louis: Mosby; 2012.
3. **Cawson**
   RA Cawson, WH Binnie, AW Barret, JM Wright. Oral Disease. 3rd ed. UK: Mosby (Harcourt Publishers Ltd.); 2001.
4. **Berkovitz**
   BKB Berkovitz, GR Holland, BJ Moxham. Oral Anatomy, Histology and Embryology. 3rd ed. Edinburgh: Elsevier; 2002.
5. **Inderbir Singh**
   I Singh. Human Embryology. 10th ed. New Delhi: Jaypee Brothers Medical Publishers Pvt. Ltd.; 2014.
6. **Arup Das**
   AK Das. Dental Anatomy and Oral Histology. Kolkata: Current Distributors; 2005.
7. emedicine.medscape.com/article/1254517-overview
8. Neville BW, Damm DD, Allen CM, Bouquot BE. Oral and Maxillofacial Pathology. 3rd ed. Philadelphia: Elsevier; 2008.
9. Rajendran R, Sivapathasundharam B. Shafer's Textbook of Oral Pathology. 7th ed. New Delhi: Elsevier; 2012.

Viva Voce Questions with Answers

1. DEVELOPMENT OF TOOTH

1. What are the different stages of tooth development?
Ans.
 i. Bud stage
 ii. Cap stage
 iii. Bell stage
 iv. Advanced bell stage
 v. Root development

2. Why are they named as such?
Ans.
• According to the shape of enamel organ (epithelial part of tooth germ)

3. In cap stage, what does enamel organ consist of?
Ans.
 i. Outer enamel epithelium
 ii. Stellate reticulum
 iii. Inner enamel epithelium

4. What is the function of stellate reticulum?
Ans. It acts as a shock absorber to support and protect delicate enamel-forming cells.

5. In bell stage, what does the enamel organ consist of?
Ans.
 i. Outer enamel epithelium
 ii. Stellate reticulum
 iii. Stratum intermedium
 iv. Inner enamel epithelium

6. What is the function of stratum intermedium?
Ans. It seems to be essential for enamel formation.

7. What is membrana preformativa?
Ans. It is the basement membrane separating the enamel organ and dental papilla, which is future dentinoenamel junction.

8. Which structures are developed from dental papilla?
Ans. Dentin and pulp

9. Which structures are developed from dental sac?
Ans. Cementum, periodontal ligament and alveolar bone

10. Enamel organ gives rise to formation of what?
Ans. Enamel

11. What are the remnants of dental lamina called as?
Ans. Cell rests of Serres

12. In which stage does the formation of hard dental tissues take place?
Ans. Advanced bell stage

13. Which hard tissue is formed first?
Ans. Dentin

14. What is Hertwig's epithelial root sheath (HERS)?
Ans. Outer enamel epithelium and inner enamel epithelium meet at future cementoenamel junction which forms HERS.

15. What is the function of HERS?
Ans. Root formation

16. What are the remnants of HERS?
Ans. Cell rests of Malassez

2. ENAMEL

1. What are the formative cells of enamel?
Ans. Ameloblasts

2. Which cells are differentiated into ameloblasts?
Ans. Inner enamel epithelial cells of enamel organ

3. What are the incremental lines in enamel?
Ans. Incremental lines of Retzius.

4. What do these lines indicate?
Ans. - Successive apposition of layers of enamel during crown formation.

5. What is neonatal line?
Ans. The line which separates the enamel formed before birth (prenatal enamel) and the enamel formed after birth (postnatal enamel). It is the accentuated incremental line of Retzius.

6. In which teeth is the neonatal line present?
Ans. In deciduous teeth and first permanent molars.

7. Which enamel is of better quality and why?
Ans. Prenatal enamel as it develops in a well-protected environment with adequate supply of all essential materials.

8. How is the dentinoenamel junction appear in ground section?
Ans. Scalloped with convexities towards the dentin.

9. What are enamel tufts?
Ans. Narrow ribbon-like structures arising from dentinoenamel junction resembling a tuft of grass.

10. What are enamel spindles?
Ans. Odontoblastic processes of dentin cross the dentinoenamel junction and extend into enamel.

11. What are enamel lamellae?
Ans. Hypocalcified structures extending from the enamel surface towards the dentinoenamel junction.

12. What are types of enamel lamellae?
Ans.
Type A – composed of poorly calcified rod segments
Type B – composed of degenerated cells
Type C – seen in erupted teeth where cracks are filled with organic matter derived from saliva

13. What are Hunter–Schreger bands?
Ans.
Alternate dark and light bands originating at dentinoenamel junction
Dark bands – diazones
Light bands – parazones

14. What is gnarled enamel?
Ans. In cuspal region, the enamel rods appear to be twisted around each other forming more complex arrangement of the rods.

15. Name the hypocalcified structures in enamel?
Ans.
  i) Incremental lines of Retzius
 ii) Neonatal line
iii) Enamel tufts
 iv) Enamel spindles
  v) Enamel lamellae
 vi) Hunter–Schreger bands

16. What are the stages in the life cycle of ameloblasts?
Ans.
i) Morphogenic; ii) Organizing; iii) Formative; iv) Maturative; v) Protective; vi) Desmolytic

17. What is the chemical composition of enamel?
Ans.
Inorganic material – 96%
Organic substance and water – 4%

3. DENTIN

1. What is the composition of dentin?
Ans.
Inorganic material – 65%
Organic material and water – 35%

2. What are the formative cells of dentin?
Ans. Odontoblasts

3. What does the dentin consist of?
Ans. Dentinal tubules

4. What do these dentinal tubules contain?
Ans. Cytoplasmic extensions of odontoblasts.

5. What is the shape of dentinal tubules?
Ans. Gentle S-shaped: starting at right angle from the pulpal surface, the first convexity of this S-shaped curvature is directed towards the apex of the root of the tooth.

6. What is peritubular dentin?
Ans. The dentin that immediately surrounds the dentinal tubules. This dentin forms the walls of the dentinal tubules.

7. What is intertubular dentin?
Ans. It is the dentin present between the zones of peritubular dentin. It forms the main body of the dentin.

8. What is predentin?
Ans. It is the unmineralized dentin present adjacent to pulp tissue.

9. What is primary dentin made up of?
Ans.
Mantle dentin
Circumpulpal dentin

10. Where is the mantle dentin present?
Ans. In the crown underlying dentinoenamel junction.

11. What is secondary dentin?
Ans. The dentin formed after root completion.

12. Where is the secondary dentin present?
Ans. It is narrow band of dentin bordering the pulp.

13. What is tertiary dentin?
Ans. The dentin formed as a reaction to trauma such as caries or restorative procedures.

14. What are the incremental lines in dentin called?
Ans. Incremental lines of von Ebner

15. What do these incremental lines indicate?
Ans. Daily rhythmic, recurrent deposition of dentin matrix as well as a hesitation in the daily formative process.

16. What are the contour lines of Owen?
Ans. Accentuated incremental lines are known as contour lines of Owen.

17. What is interglobular dentin?

Ans. Sometimes mineralization of dentin takes place in the form of small globules which fail to coalesce into a homogenous mass. This forms the zones of hypomineralization between the globules. These zones are known as interglobular dentin.

18. What is Tomes' granular layer?

Ans. A granular zone in the root dentin adjacent to cementum.

19. What are the theories of pain transmission through dentin?

Ans.
  (i) Direct neural stimulation
 (ii) Fluid or hydrodynamic theory
(iii) Transduction theory

20. What are dead tracts?

Ans. In dried ground section of normal dentin, the odontoblast processes disintegrate and empty tubules are filled with air, they appear black in transmitted light and white in reflected light.

21. What is sclerotic or transparent dentin?

Ans. It is the area where lumen of the dentinal tubule is obliterated with mineral which appears transparent or light in transmitted light and dark in reflected light.

4. PULP

1. What are the different zones in the pulp at periphery?

Ans.
  (i) Odontoblasts
 (ii) Cell-free zone (Weil's zone)
(iii) Cell-rich zone (of undifferentiated mesenchymal cells and fibroblasts)

2. What are the shapes of odontoblasts at different levels in pulp?

Ans.
Tall columnar in crown
Cuboidal in the middle of the root
Ovoid or spindle shaped close to the apex of tooth

3. What are the defence cells in the pulp?

Ans. Histiocytes or macrophages, dendritic cells, mast cells, plasma cells, neutrophils, eosinophils, basophils, lymphocytes and monocytes

4. What are the functions of pulp?

Ans.
Inductive
Formative
Nutritive
Protective
Defensive

5. What are pulp stones (denticles)?

Ans. Nodular calcified masses in the pulp.

6. What are the types of pulp stones?

Ans.

According to structure – True pulp stones, False pulp stones

According to the relation to the dentin of the tooth – Free pulp stone, Attached pulp stone, Embedded pulp stones

7. What is the difference between true and false pulp stones?

Ans. True pulp stones are similar to dentin in structure (presence of dentinal tubules with odontoblast on their surface). False pulp stones do not contain dentinal tubules but appear as concentric layers of calcified tissue.

8. What are the diffuse calcifications?

Ans. Irregular calcific deposits in the pulp usually found in the root

6. PERIODONTAL LIGAMENT

1. Name the principal fibres of periodontal ligament

Ans.

Alveolar crest group

Horizontal group

Oblique group

Apical group

Interradicular group in multirooted teeth

2. What are Sharpey's fibres?

Ans. Collagen fibres embedded into cementum or alveolar bone are known as Sharpey's fibres.

3. What are functions of periodontal ligament?

Ans.

Supportive

Sensory

Nutritive

Homeostatic

Eruptive

4. What are the cells present in the periodontal ligament?

Ans.

Synthetic cells – fibroblasts, osteoblasts, cementoblasts

Resorptive cells – fibroblasts, osteoclasts, cementoclasts

Progenitor cells

Epithelial rests of Malassez

Defence cells – mast cells, macrophages, eosinophils

5. What are cementicles?

Ans. Calcified bodies found in the periodontal ligament are called as cementicles.

7. ALVEOLAR BONE

1. What are the functions of bone?

Ans.

It provides shape and support to the body.

It provides site of attachment for tendons and muscles.

It protects vital organs of the body.

It serves as a storage site for minerals and provides the medium for development and storage of blood cells.

2. How are the bones classified?
Ans.
According to shape – long, flat and irregular
According to mode of development – endochondral and intramembranous bones
According to microscopic structure – mature bones (compact and cancellous) and immature bone (woven bone)

3. What is Haversian system?
Ans. Haversian canal with concentric lamellae is known as Haversian system or osteon.

4. What is reversal line?
Ans. Reversal lines are highly irregular, strongly basophilic lines formed by the scalloped outline of the Howship's lacunae and mark the limit of bone erosion prior to the formation of osteon.

5. What is resting line?
Ans. Resting line is a more regular line which denotes the period of rest during the formation of bone.

6. What are Volkmann canals?
Ans. Adjacent Haversian canals interconnected by channels that contain blood vessels are known as Volkmann canals.

7. What are the formative cells of bone?
Ans. Osteoblasts

8. What are osteoclasts?
Ans. Osteoclasts are bone-resorbing cells. These are large, multinucleated cell which lie in resorption bays known as Howship's lacunae.

9. What is woven bone?
Ans. It is the immature bone characterized by intertwined collagen fibres oriented in many directions. As it is formed rapidly, many osteocytes are incorporated within it.

10. What is alveolar process?
Ans. It is that part of the maxilla and mandible that forms and supports the socket of the teeth.

11. What is bundle bone?
Ans. It is the bone in which the principal fibres of periodontal ligament are anchored.

12. What is alveolar bone proper?
Ans. It is the bone which forms the inner wall of the socket. It is perforated by many openings that carry branches of the intra-alveolar nerves and blood vessels into the periodontal ligament and so are called as cribriform plate.

8. ORAL MUCOUS MEMBRANE

1. What is the classification of oral mucosa?
Ans.
Masticatory mucosa
Lining mucosa
Specialized mucosa

2. Which areas of oral mucosa are covered by masticatory mucosa?
Ans. Gingiva and hard palate

3. Which areas of oral mucosa are covered by lining mucosa?
Ans. Lip, cheek, vestibular fornix, alveolar mucosa, floor of mouth and soft palate

4. Which area of oral mucosa is covered by specialized mucosa?
Ans. Dorsum of tongue

5. What are the functions of oral mucosa?
Ans.
Defence
Lubrication
Sensory
Protection

6. What is basement membrane?
Ans. It is the interface between the epithelium and connective tissue.

7. Which is the special stain for basement membrane?
Ans. Periodic acid–Schiff stain (PAS stain), where it takes a magenta colour.

8. What are the different layers in oral epithelium in stratified squamous keratinized epithelium?
Ans.
Stratum basale
Stratum spinosum
Stratum granulosum
Stratum corneum

9. What is stratum germinativum?
Ans. Basal cells and parabasal spinous cells are known as stratum germinativum.

10. What are the granules in stratum granulosum? Which colour do they have with haemotoxylin and eosin stain?
Ans. Keratohyalin granules are present in stratum granulosum and they show blue colour.

11. Name the nonkeratinocytes present in oral mucosa?
Ans.
Melanocytes
Langerhans cells
Merkel's cells
Other cells such as lymphocytes and polymorphonuclear leukocytes

12. What are the different layers in oral epithelium in nonkeratinized stratified squamous epithelium?
Ans.
Stratum basale
Stratum intermedium
Stratum superficiale

13. What is present in the connective tissue of anterolateral zone of hard palate?
Ans. Adipose tissue

14. What is present in the connective tissue of posterolateral zone of hard palate?
Ans. Mucous glands

15. What is the epithelium of gingiva?
Ans. It is stratified squamous epithelium which is keratinized or nonkeratinized, most often parakeratinized.

16. Name the fibres of gingival ligament.
Ans.
Dentogingival
Alveologingival
Circular
Dentoperiosteal

17. What are the different papillae present on the tongue?
Ans.
Filiform
Fungiform
Circumvallate
Foliate

18. Which papillae do not contain taste buds?
Ans. Filiform

19. What is the colour of fungiform papillae?
Ans. Reddish

20. Where are the circumvallate papillae present?
Ans. They are present anterior to sulcus terminalis (V-shaped terminal sulcus between body and base of the tongue). They are 8–10 in number.

21. The ducts of which gland open into the trough of circumvallate papillae?
Ans. von Ebner's gland

22. What is the nature of these glands?
Ans. Serous

23. What are taste buds?
Ans. Taste buds are small ovoid or barrel-shaped intraepithelial organs extending from basal lamina to the surface of the epithelium.

24. What is gingival sulcus?
Ans. Gingival sulcus is the space between the inner aspect of gingiva and tooth.

25. What is the normal depth of gingival sulcus?
Ans. The normal depth of gingival sulcus is around 2 mm.

9. SALIVARY GLANDS

1. What are serous cells?
Ans. Serous cells are pyramidal with broad base resting on the basement membrane with spherical nucleus at the basal region and secretory granules in the apical cytoplasm.

2. What are these secretory granules?
Ans. Zymogen granules

3. What are mucous cells?
Ans. In mucous cells the apex appears empty and the nucleus and a thin rim of cytoplasm is compressed against the base of the cells.

4. How does the mucous secretion differ from serous secretion?
Ans.
- Mucous secretion has little or no enzymatic activity; it is mainly for lubrication and protection for oral tissues.
- The ratio of carbohydrate to protein is greater; larger amount of sialic acid is present.

5. What are myoepithelial cells?
Ans. Myoepithelial cells are stellate or spider-like cells which branching processes that embrace the secretory and intercalated duct cells.

6. What is the other name of myoepithelial cells?
Ans. Basket cells

7. Where are these located?
Ans. They are located around the terminal secretory unit and intercalated duct cells between the base of these cells and the basement membrane.

8. What are the functions of myoepithelial cells?
Ans.
- Accelerate the initial outflow of saliva from the acini
- Reduce the luminal volume
- Support the underlying parenchyma and reduce the back permeation of fluid
- Help salivary flow to overcome in peripheral resistance of ducts
- Contribute to secretory pressure in the acini or duct

9. What is the duct system of salivary glands?
Ans.
Intercalated ducts
Striated duct and excretory ducts

10. Name the intralobular ducts.
Ans. Intercalated and striated ducts

11. Name the interlobular duct.
Ans. Excretory duct

12. Name the major salivary glands.
Ans.
Parotid gland
Submandibular gland
Sublingual gland

13. What is the nature of parotid gland?
Ans. Pure serous in nature

14. What is the name of the excretory duct of parotid gland? Where does it open?
Ans. Stensen's duct; it opens at the buccal mucosa opposite maxillary second molar.

15. What is the name of excretory duct of submandibular gland? Where does it open?
Ans. Wharton's duct; it opens at the sublingual papillae lateral to the lingual foramen.

16. What is the nature of the submandibular gland?
Ans. Mixed gland with predominantly serous units

17. What is the name of the excretory duct of sublingual glands? Where does it open?
Ans. Bartholin's duct; it opens with or near the submandibular duct.

18. What is the nature of sublingual gland?
Ans. Mixed gland which is predominantly mucous in nature.

19. What are the minor salivary glands on the tongue located near to the apex of the tongue?
Ans. Glands of Blandin and Nuhn

20. What is the composition of saliva?
Ans.
99% or more–water
1% or less–inorganic ions, secretory proteins and other substances

21. What is the pH of whole saliva?
Ans. 6.4–7.4

22. What is the total volume of saliva secreted daily in humans?
Ans. 750–1000 mL

23. What are the functions of saliva?
Ans.
• Protection of oral cavity and oral environment
• Digestion
• Mastication
• Taste perception
• Speech
• Tissue repair
• Excretion

24. What are demilunes?
Ans. Sometimes mucous acini have crescent-shaped covering of serous cells, these are known as demilunes.

10. MAXILLARY SINUS

1. What is maxillary sinus?
Ans. It is a pneumatic space located inside the body of maxilla.

2. How is the lining epithelium of maxillary sinus?
Ans. Pseudostratified ciliated columnar epithelium

3. What are Goblet cells?
Ans. Column-shaped cells found among epithelial lining of respiratory tract which secrete mucous.

4. What are the functions of maxillary sinus?

Ans.

Humidification and warming of inspired air

Resonance of voice

Lightening of skull weight

Enhancement of faciocranial resistance to mechanical shock

Production of bactericidal lysozyme to nasal cavity

ORAL PATHOLOGY

11. BENIGN AND MALIGNANT TUMOURS OF THE ORAL CAVITY

1. What are koilocytes?

Ans. Human papilloma virus (HPV) altered epithelial cells with perinuclear clear spaces and nuclear pyknosis.

2. What is papilloma?

Ans. It is a benign tumour of epithelial tissue origin.

3. What is leukoplakia?

Ans. It is the most common potentially malignant lesion defined as a predominantly white lesion of the oral mucosa that cannot be characterized as any other definable lesion.

4. What are the histological features of epithelial dysplasia?

Ans.

- Loss of polarity of basal cells
- Increased nuclear cytoplasmic ratio
- Drop-shaped rete processes
- Irregular epithelial stratification
- Increased number of mitotic figures
- Presence of mitotic figures in the superficial half of the epithelium
- Cellular pleomorphism
- Nuclear hyperchromatism
- Enlarged nucleoli
- Reduction of cellular cohesion
- Keratinization of single cells or cell groups in the prickle layer

5. What are the grades of epithelial dysplasia?

Ans.

- Mild epithelial dysplasia – if the dysplastic features are seen in basal and parabasal layer.
- Moderate epithelial dysplasia – if the dysplastic features are seen from basal cell layer to mid-portion of spinous cell layer.
- Severe epithelial dysplasia – if the dysplastic features are seen from basal cell layer to a level above the midpoint of the epithelium.

6. What is carcinoma in situ (intraepithelial carcinoma)?

Ans. It is a condition characterized by top to bottom epithelial dysplasia, i.e. dysplastic features extending from basal layer to the surface of the epithelium.

7. What is oral submucous fibrosis?

Ans. It is a chronic, progressive, scarring potentially malignant disorder in which the oral mucosa becomes fibrotic, and progressively there is trismus.

8. What is squamous cell carcinoma?
Ans. It is the most common malignant neoplasm of epithelial tissue origin.

9. What are the grades of squamous cell carcinoma?
Ans.
- Well-differentiated squamous cell carcinoma
- Moderately differentiated squamous cell carcinoma
- Poorly differentiated squamous cell carcinoma

According to the degree to which the tumour resembles a parent tissue, i.e. squamous epithelium and production of its normal product, i.e. keratin.

10. What is verrucous carcinoma?
Ans. It is a low-grade variant of oral squamous cell carcinoma.

11. What are the histopathological features of verrucous carcinoma?
Ans.
- Exophytic overgrowth of well-differentiated stratified squamous epithelium with papillary surface
- Wide elongated rete ridges with pushing borders
- Cleft-like spaces with a thick layer of parakeratin extending deeply into the lesion (parakeratin plugging)
- Intact basement membrane
- Intense chronic inflammatory cell infiltration in the connective tissue

12. What is malignant melanoma?
Ans. It is a malignant neoplasm of melanocytes.

13. What is fibroma?
Ans. It is most common benign connective tissue tumour of the oral cavity.

14. What is aneurysmal bone cyst?
Ans. It is a rare benign intraosseous nonepithelial lined cystic lesion.

15. What is histopathology of aneurysmal bone cyst?
Ans.
- Blood-filled cystic spaces of variable sizes which are not lined by endothelium
- Multinucleated giant cells within the connective tissue stroma
- Trabeculae of osteoid or woven bone
- Areas of haemosiderin deposits frequently seen

16. Name the benign tumours of nerve tissue origin.
Ans. Traumatic neuroma, neurofibroma, neurilemmoma

17. What is the characteristic histopathological pattern seen in fibrosarcoma?
Ans. Herringbone pattern.

18. What is the characteristic histopathologic feature of osteosarcoma?
Ans. Presence of tumour osteoid (osteoid formed by malignant osteoblasts)

12. TUMOURS OF SALIVARY GLANDS

1. Which is the most common benign salivary gland tumour?
Ans. Pleomorphic adenoma

2. Which is the most common characteristic histopathologic pattern of adenoid cystic carcinoma?
Ans. Cribriform pattern

3. What are the histological grades of mucoepidermoid carcinoma?
Ans. Low grade, intermediate grade and high grade, depending on amount of cyst formation, degree of cytologic atypia and relative numbers of mucous, epidermoid and intermediate cells

13. ODONTOGENIC CYSTS

1. What are the characteristic histopathological features of odontogenic keratocyst?
Ans. Cystic lumen lined by
a) Uniform thickness of stratified squamous epithelium about 6–10 cells thick.
b) Parakeratinized corrugated or wrinkled appearance of surface layer.
c) Well-defined prominent palisaded polarized layer of cuboidal or columnar cells resembling picket fence or tombstone appearance.
d) The fibrous connective tissue wall often shows presence of satellite or daughter cyst, cords or islands of odontogenic epithelium.

2. Which cyst is always associated with the crown unerupted or impacted tooth?
Ans. Dentigerous cyst

3. Which cyst has the potential to undergo ameloblastomatous changes?
Ans. Dentigerous cyst

4. What are the criteria suggested by Vickers and Gorlin for ameloblastomatous changes in dentigerous cyst?
Ans.
• Hyperchromatism of basal cell nuclei.
• Palisading with polarization of basal cells
• Cytoplasmic vacuolization with intercellular spacing of lining epithelium.

5. Which cyst shows presence of ghost cells?
Ans. Calcifying odontogenic cyst or Gorlin cyst

6. What are Ghost cells?
Ans. Larger epithelial cells with eosinophilic cytoplasm and loss of nuclei with preservation of basic cell outline.

14. ODONTOGENIC TUMOURS

1. What are the histological subtypes of ameloblastoma?
Ans. (i) Follicular ameloblastoma; (ii) Plexiform ameloblastoma; (iii) Acanthomatous ameloblastoma; (iv) Granular cell ameloblastoma; (v) Basal cell ameloblastoma; (vi) Desmoplastic ameloblastoma

2. Which is the most common histological subtype?
Ans. Follicular ameloblastoma

3. In which type of ameloblastoma, cyst formation is common?
Ans. Follicular ameloblastoma

4. What is the histopathology of follicular ameloblastoma?
Ans. It consists of many small islands of epithelial cells resembling enamel organ in a mature fibrous connective tissue stroma. These epithelial islands consist of peripheral layer of cuboidal or columnar ameloblast-like cells showing reversal polarity and enclose a central core of stellate reticulum-like tissue.

5. How are the tumour cells arranged in plexiform ameloblastoma?
Ans. Tumour cells are arranged in long, interconnecting strands or cords of odontogenic epithelium.

6. What is the histopathology of acanthomatous ameloblastoma?
Ans. The central portions of epithelial islands of follicular ameloblastoma resembling stellate reticulum-like tissue undergo squamous metaplasia.

7. What is the histopathology of granular cell ameloblastoma?
Ans. There is a transformation of cytoplasm of stellate reticulum-like tissue to granular cells.

8. What is the colour of these granules? What are these granules?
Ans. These are lysosomal aggregates which are eosinophilic in colour.

9. Which is the most aggressive type of ameloblastoma?
Ans. Granular cell ameloblastoma

10. Which is the least common type of ameloblastoma?
Ans. Basal cell ameloblastoma which resembles basal carcinoma of skin

11. What are histopathological groups of unicystic ameloblastoma?
Ans.
 (i) Luminal unicystic ameloblastoma
 (ii) Intraluminal unicystic ameloblastoma
(iii) Mural unicystic ameloblastoma

12. What is the other name for calcifying epithelial odontogenic tumour?
Ans. Pindborg tumour

13. What are Liesegang rings? In which odontogenic tumour are these seen?
Ans. Liesegang rings are calcifications in the form of concentric rings. They are seen in calcifying epithelial odontogenic tumour.

14. What is the histopathology of ameloblastic fibroma?
Ans. There is proliferation of epithelial and mesenchymal components without formation of enamel and dentin. The epithelial component resembles dental lamina of early tooth development and the mesenchymal component resembles dental papilla.

15. What are odontomas?
Ans. These are the most common types of mixed odontogenic tumours and considered as hamartomas. In these, both the epithelial and mesenchymal cells undergo complete differentiation to form enamel and dentin.

16. What are the types of odontomas?
Ans.
 (i) Complex composite odontoma
 (ii) Compound composite odontoma

17. Why these are called composite odontomas?
Ans. As the lesion is composed of more than one type of tissue.

18. What is the difference between compound composite and complex composite odontoma?
Ans. Compound odontomas have a considerable resemblance to normal teeth whereas complex odontomas have no morphological similarity to normal teeth.

15. REGRESSIVE ALTERATIONS OF TEETH

1. Define attrition.
Ans. Attrition is defined as the physiologic wearing away of a tooth as a result of tooth-to-tooth contact as in mastication.

2. Define abrasion.
Ans. Abrasion is the pathologic wearing away of a tooth substance through some abnormal mechanical process.

3. What is pulp fibrosis?
Ans. It is a regressive change in ageing pulp with deposition of bundles of collagen fibres and diffuse fibrillar components.

4. What are pulp stones?
Ans. Nodular calcified masses in the pulp.

5. What are types of pulp stones?
Ans.
• According to structure – True pulp stones, False pulp stones
• According to the relation to the dentin of the tooth – Free pulp stone, Attached pulp stone, Embedded pulp stones

6. What is the difference between true and false pulp stones?
Ans. True pulp stones are similar to dentin in structure (presence of dentinal tubules with odontoblast on their surface). False pulp stones do not contain dentinal tubules but appear as concentric layers of calcified tissue.

7. What are diffuse calcifications?
Ans. Diffuse calcifications are amorphous dystrophic calcifications which appear as irregular linear strands of calcific deposits.

16. BACTERIAL AND MYCOTIC INFECTIONS

1. What are streptococci?
Ans. Gram-positive ovoid or spherical cocci arranged in chains

2. What are staphylococci?
Ans. Gram-positive spherical cocci arranged in grape-like clusters

3. Name the causative microorganism of tuberculosis?
Ans. Mycobacterium tuberculosis

4. Which stain is used to stain these microorganisms?
Ans. Ziehl–Neelsen stain where these microorganisms appear as bright red bacilli

5. What is the histopathology of tuberculous granuloma?
Ans. It is a circumscribed area of infection with central caseous necrosis surrounded by epitheloid histiocytes, lymphocytes and Langhans giant cells.

6. Name the causative microorganism of leprosy?
Ans. Mycobacterium leprae

7. Which stain is used to stain Corynebacterium diphtheriae?
Ans. Albert stain

8. Name the causative microorganism of actinomycosis.
Ans. Actinomyces israelii

9. What are sulphur granules?
Ans. In actinomycosis, the abscesses discharging pus usually containing yellowish flecks are sulphur granules. These are colonies of Actinomyces.

10. What is the characteristic histologic appearance of Actinomyces colony?
Ans. Ray fungus appearance

11. Name the infection caused by Candida albicans.
Ans. Candidiasis (candidosis, moniliasis, thrush)

12. What is pyogenic granuloma?
Ans. It is a common tumour-like growth of the oral cavity as a response of the tissues to a nonspecific infection.

17. DENTAL CARIES

1. What is the shape of the pit and fissure caries?
Ans. A triangular or cone-shaped lesion with the base towards the dentinoenamel junction and apex at the outer surface.

2. What are the different histological zones of enamel caries?
Ans. Starting from inner advancing front of the lesion, the zones are (i) Translucent zone, (ii) Dark zone, (iii) Body of lesion, (iv) Surface zone.

3. What is liquefaction foci described by Miller?
Ans. In advanced dentinal caries, there is a focal coalescence and breakdown of few dentinal tubules which form a tiny liquefaction foci described by Miller. It appears as an ovoid area of destruction filled with necrotic debris and runs parallel to the direction of tubules.

4. What are transverse clefts?
Ans. The extension of caries process along the lateral branches of dentinal tubules and along the matrix fibres leads to formation of transverse clefts which are at right angle to the dentinal tubules.

5. What are the various zones of carious dentin?
Ans.
Zone 1: Zone of fatty degeneration of odontoblast process
Zone 2: Zone of dentinal sclerosis
Zone 3: Zone of decalcification of dentin

Zone 4: Zone of bacterial invasion of decalcified but intact dentin
Zone 5: Zone of decomposed dentin

18. DISEASES OF PULP AND PERIAPICAL TISSUES

1. What is chronic hyperplastic pulpitis?
Ans. It is a type of chronic pulpitis occurring in children and young adults with high pulp tissue resistance and reactivity.

2. What is the histopathology of chronic hyperplastic pulpitis?
Ans. There is a formation of granulation tissue covered by stratified squamous epithelium and this mass of tissue protrudes from the pulp chamber into the carious lesion.

3. What is periapical granuloma?
Ans. It is a localized mass of chronic granulation tissue at the apex of the root of the nonvital tooth as a response to infection.

4. How does the periapical granuloma undergo cystic changes?
Ans. There is a proliferation of epithelial rests of Malassez incorporated within the periapical granuloma in an irregular pattern. Due to continued proliferation, there is increase in epithelial mass by division of basal cells on the periphery. Thus, the cells in the central part of the mass do not get nutrition. They degenerate, become necrotic and liquefy. This forms an epithelial lined cystic cavity filled with fluid.

5. What are Rushton bodies?
Ans. Tiny, linear or arc-shaped bodies seen in the lining epithelium of radicular cyst (or in cysts with inflammation). These bodies are amorphous in structure, eosinophilic in reaction and brittle in nature.

6. What is sequestrum?
Ans. It is a fragment of necrotic (dead) bone which is separated from adjacent vital bone.

7. What is involucrum?
Ans. Fragments of necrotic bone may be surrounded by new vital bone known as involucrum.

19. DISEASES OF BONES

1. What is fibrous dysplasia?
Ans. It is a developmental tumour-like condition that is characterized by replacement of normal bone by an excessive proliferation of cellular fibrous connective tissue with formation of secondary metaplastic bone.

2. What is the characteristic shape of bony trabeculae in fibrous dysplasia?
Ans. Irregular, slender, Chinese letter pattern (C-shaped)

3. What is Paget disease?
Ans. It is a chronic progressive disorder characterized by abnormal and disorganized resorption and deposition of bone.

4. What is histopathological appearance of Paget disease?
Ans. Jigsaw puzzle or mosaic appearance

5. What is the other name for Paget disease?
Ans. Osteitis deformans

20. DISEASES OF SKIN

1. What are civatte bodies?
Ans. Degenerating keratinocytes are seen as homogenous, eosinophilic globules at epithelium and connective tissue interface in oral lichen planus.

2. What is acantholysis?
Ans. The cells of spinous cell layers lose their attachments, which is called acantholysis (seen in pemphigus).

3. What are Tzanck cells?
Ans. The cells of spinous cell layer lose their attachment, these loose cells become rounded in shape and cytoplasm around nucleus contracts with swelling of the nuclei and hyperchromatic staining. These cells are known as Tzanck cells.

4. Which vesicle or bulla formation is seen in pemphigus?
Ans. Intraepithelial vesicle or bulla formation

5. Which vesicle or bulla formation is seen in benign mucous membrane pemphigoid?
Ans. Subepithelial vesicle or bulla formation.

6. Which syndrome is associated with severe form of Erythema multiforme?
Ans. Stevens–Johnson Syndrome.

21. CYSTS OF NONODONTOGENIC ORIGIN

1. What is the other name for nasopalatine duct cyst?
Ans. Incisive canal cyst

2. What is the histopathology of thyroglossal duct cyst?
Ans. Cystic cavity is lined by stratified squamous, ciliated columnar or intermediate transition-type epithelium. The underlying connective tissue wall shows presence of thyroid tissue, small patches of lymphoid tissue and mucous glands.

3. What is mucocele?
Ans. It is a nonodontogenic cyst of salivary gland origin.

4. Which is the most common site for mucocele?
Ans. Lower lip.

5. How have mucocele been classified?
Ans.
a) Extravasation mucocele and b) Retention mucocele (true retention cyst)

6. Which is the most common type?
Ans. Extravasation mucocele

Index